BREATH, SLEEP, THE HEART, AND LIFE

BReath, sleep, the heaRt, and life

THE REVOLUTIONARY HEALTH YOGA OF PUNDIT ACHARYA

The Laughing Man Series of Classic Spiritual Literature

THE DAWN HORSE PRESS
LOWER LAKE, CALIFORNIA

THE DAWN HORSE PRESS
P. O. Box 677
Lower Lake, California 95457

This book is a compilation of four works by Pundit Acharya: *You Haven't Slept* (Copyright 1955 by Prana Press), *This Precious Heart* (Copyright 1958 by Prana Press), *Internal Respiration* (Copyright 1954 by Prana Press), *Breath Is Life* (Copyright 1951 by Prana Press). For permission to reprint Pundit Acharya's original works we gratefully acknowledge Prana Press (Temple of Yogas, Inc.), The Acharyan, 265 River Road, Nyack, New York 10960.

International Standard Book Number:
0-913922-09-9
Library of Congress Card Catalog Number:
74-24306

Printed in the United States of America

CONTENTS

ACKNOWLEDGEMENTS

We gratefully acknowledge Prana Press (Temple of Yogas, Inc.); The Acharyan, 265 River Road, Nyack, New York, for permission to reprint these works of Dr. Pundit Acharya.

Acknowledgement to *Paraplay Magazine,* Prana Press, Nyack, New York for reprint of "Your Ageless Cells."

Cover design: from an original wood block print by Hasui (1884-1957), "Morning sea of Uikuni, Shiribeshi." Printed 1933. Published by Watanabe Shozaburo, Tokyo.

PREFACE

Dr. Acharya was born a Vedic Brahmin of India. He gave up high caste and privilege to tend cholera victims in the streets while still a boy. As a teenager he was an editor for *The New Age* in Calcutta when he led the fight for India's independence in his editorials. He attended Columbia University and the University of Iowa, and he lived American life in all its phases. He initiated milk drives for undernourished children in Chicago and he was a Red Cross Lecturer during World War I.

Poet, playwright, and composer, he was editor of *Superman*, a magazine sponsored by G.B. Shaw and Rabindranath Tagore. Dr. Acharya founded the first Yoga Research School in the United States, reinterpreting the Yogas in terms of neuro-bio-electronics. He demonstrated the Acharyan Methods at the Harvard Psychological Clinic. The Temple of Yogas, Inc., founded by Dr. Acharya, is the repository for his studies.

Dr. Pundit Acharya's forty years of research along empirical lines with men and women in all walks of life resulted in the development of a new type of exercise: tending toward effortless effort in gentle paraplays of release and bioplays of life.

These plays of life are joyful plays of the biotic being in infinitely slow, graduated motion—slower than a slow motion camera. When practiced with *feeling* of the bodily sensation reported to the brain—true sensory perception—these paraplays tend to arrest motor degeneration and release the honeyed secretions of the body in a pleasant flow of life without jerks or creases.

The bioplays of life to activate the cells of the body and vitalize the protoplasm are also paraplays of release. They are in reality replays of our biotic being along the biological path of evolution with emphasis on bi-lateral development.

There are hundreds of these exercises and some are varied many times, so that they do not become automatic as in walking. It is the quality of the exercise rather than the technique which is important.

Here exercise becomes play, work becomes play, life becomes play, wherein at last we begin to escape from gravity into the realm of gravitation. In other words, we shall have a flowing along with life instead of constant struggle against it.

The Acharyan Method is a study of the protoplasm of man in terms of its neuro-bio-electronic potential. It differs from all other methods of exercises as it lays stress upon the play of the para-sympathetic system in physiological movements based upon the biotic being and the protoplasm itself. It involves a definite sensation of feeling (the most delicate form of perception), rather than volition and muscular exertion. It requires infinite slowness in the exercises, gentle mouth breathing by sagging of the jaw, and bending of the neck, together with the generation of a new hormone called *Amiya* and *the Smile* in the literature of the Institute.

Yoga Research Institute.

INTRODUCTION

YOUR AGELESS CELLS

By G.A. Brooks

General Secretary
Yoga Research Institute

Modern science has discovered that the essential material of our being is the protoplasm and that the cells of which our protoplasm is composed are ageless,* that it is the whole man with his framework which degenerates and dies, and that this decay begins practically at maturity, the age of 21, or earlier.

The corollary is evident, that either the functional specialization of the cell groups is inadequate, or there is not complete coordination among these cell groups in the human body. Perhaps both. At any rate, we know one thing for sure, and that is whether science keeps us alive until the age of 67 on the average or until 77, as it seems likely to do, we are far from being really alive. Already at maturity we begin to lose our flexibility. The flame of youth—daring, supple, ready for anything and everything—begins to die into a flickering spark, and by 40, though still on our feet, the process of degeneration exceeds the rate of regeneration. In plain words, we are more dead than alive.

In earlier times it is recorded that men have lived to the age of three hundred or more years. We do not know whether they were still young at heart at that age or not, but we must presume that their arteries were still good and they had not yet started to die at the age of 21 if they lived to the age of 300. In those days there was also a science of agelessness known to the sages of India. These

*N. Y. *Herald Tribune,* October 17, 1954

ix

sages invented a system of bodily training—a method of unison designed to keep man healthy and young and at the peak of physical power, regardless of the length of years.

Beginning with a system of bodily movements repeating the animate stages of existence, a blueprint of all the organs and glands with breathing techniques for perfect functioning of each, and a technique of sensitization and control of all these organs, it led finally to a supersonic state of brain matter, where at last the perfect being could contact and condition matter. This supersonic state of being is the divine majesty in every man awaiting its time of unfoldment.

Man shall be placed back upon his throne. This was the mission of my teacher when he came to America—to rediscover the meaning of this science and reinterpret it to the world in the light of modern practical sciences. Many times in the face of great discouragements and continual misunderstanding, he wondered if it were possible for people to learn these precious things in the midst of the world, and then perhaps he remembered his own words of prophecy: *Physics shall find the subtle stages of matter. Medicine shall be the knowledge of life. Science shall be understanding.* These were pure prophecy but in the same book* one found the story of cell memory, adrenal-thyroid drunkenness, and other physiological facts in a language strange indeed to us.

Along with hundreds of students from many parts of the world and all walks of life, I became a student of the science of being along empirical lines under this great teacher, Pundit Acharya. Among these students engaged in this scientific research were many doctors who were interested in knowing firsthand, from a descendant of one of these sages, about this science so long covered up by mystical allusions and metaphysical speculation.

However there was nothing mysterious in this school—only physiological charts of the body and a blackboard. The first thing we learned was that we were not studying metaphysics but rather a stage of physics which analytical science had not penetrated. In a world of mechanical super-science stopped short by ever-advancing new diseases, at a stage where people were willing to believe in

A Strange Language

all kinds of mind cure and mind powers, it was strange to hear from this sage that the secret of life was not mind over matter but mind *of* matter. Here was pure science and a scientific method. Any man could know it—if he had the patience to study and work with it. There were no miracles. Nature did not need miracles. They only seemed miracles because we did not know the laws of their manifestation as yet.

One author, the writer of a best-seller, had written to our teacher and said: "I'll be d––d if I'll sit down cross-legged and contemplate my navel." This expresses pretty well the state of our understanding at that time and of pretty much the whole world as regards this particular science of being, and would be still today were it not for the many researchers in the field who have come to know the meaning of this science in their own lives and have devoted their lives to passing it on.

In the forty years that our teacher gave lectures and classes throughout the country, he never said a word about the beliefs of India. He never told us what to do or what not to do. He only told us the method by which we would discover the truth for ourselves and awaken our own knowledge by the cell memory within us. It was only by a *physiological* method that we would come at last to true perception. Above all, the Pundit taught us never to take anything for granted and never to take anyone's word for anything—even his, until we had experimented on ourselves to find the truth. *To know the thing one must* BE *the thing.*

We learned that *there were no accidents in the universe—that whatever is, is of necessity.* God does not make mistakes. He represents inviolable law. Even God cannot set His own law aside. This is a hard philosophy. Anyone could see that here was a scientific attitude without doubt. Inviolable laws. Immutable God. Imperishable matter. *Spirituality is such a rare flower, it can grow only on the richest soil of material well-being.* This material well-being did not mean accumulation of possessions but the richest manifestation of matter of which the human being is the last and greatest evolution of all capable of reaching out through endless universes to touch the hand of God. America with her freedom-loving soul, said Pundit Acharya, was the matrix, where the new manifestation of spirit in finer and finer stages of matter would take place.

Here is a slight picture of the wealth of opportunity, the great gift that was ours as students to sit at the feet of such a master of life. But we Americans are a practical people. This was a science we were studying and we wanted to know the practical details. Our teacher was even more practical. He gave us so many techniques and methods that it took us fifteen years to work with them and begin to understand their meaning. Many of us who came were sick bodily and mentally, others just chronically ailing, and some given up as hopeless and incurable by their doctors. There were those too just seeking good health and happiness, others a new mastery of life.

Treatment of the human body belongs to the doctors; if the doctors who are specialists do not know, nobody knows, said our teacher. As students we had to have a working knowledge of physiology, chemistry and physics—better still, experience in a psycho-physics laboratory if possible. How else would we be able to observe correctly all the physiological detail? With this basic knowledge of our bodies, we could use the tools Pundit Acharya gave us to experiment with: procedures to the immediate end of a healthier and happier body, and the ultimate end of a coordinated being—tuned up as it were to the nth power.

We began our research along practical lines by doing different kinds of bodily movements as are taught in the gymnasiums and schools of both the West and the East. We found that all of these exercises required tenseness in some part of the body with consequent over-exertion and quick fatigue. These ordinary forms of exercise demonstrated a known law of physics: if one meets resistance with resistance by exerting force, the result can only be exhaustion leading eventually to decay and final death. It is only a question of degree as the No. 1 killer in the modern world, heart disease, will testify.

We went also to Nature to find a key. We watched the babies and young animals in natural surroundings. We watched the cat and dog in the kitten and puppy stage. We found the animals move every which way—turn and twist and stretch and yawn lazily, languorously even, and when they fight as youngsters, they do it playfully. It's just a tussle.

We saw that the babies explore everything. They crawl on the floor, wiggle and squirm, and try to put their toes in their mouth. They move every part of their body in every possible direction, continually extending their mobility—easily, without undue strain. As they moved, their mouths were always slightly open and they bubbled with joy as they played, while we, the stiff older ones, watched them.

At the same time, we studied people practicing the usual forms of muscular exercise, and we noticed how their eyes were strained, their jaws set, their faces flushed and their breath irregular. They were almost always out of breath when they stopped exercising. It was not a pretty picture. They did not look happy except when they finished, which seemed like the relief that comes from beating your head against a wall and then stopping.

The conclusion was inescapable. We are happy, healthy human beings—in the words of the popular song "by doing just what comes naturally!" in the way of bodily movement.

What was the thing that made the babies and young animals so happy in their bodily movements? There was one thing both had in common as they moved, the feeling of play—a meaningless joy or foolish feeling. The young animals didn't really fight. They just played at fighting.

So now we made more experiments on ourselves. We did the same movements in a sense of play and then we slowed them down to such slow motion that the body almost seemed to move itself. We kept our lower jaw relaxed with slightly imparted lips, like the babies, as we did these movements, and we kept our head out of it. That is, we became as little children, with our brain half awake. We dropped all thought, all imagination and *felt* the sensation of our body as we moved slowly, delicately, rhythmically. Immediately we found ourselves feeling pleasant, joyful—happy without reason. Our body felt happy. Apparently the tiny animal cells of our body loved such gentle movement, for they had immediately reported through their telegraph nerve system a lovely sensation of pleasure to our brain.

Having studied physiology in school, we now restudied it and found that our nervous system was really dual. In the ordinary type of muscular exercise we had observed that one part of the nervous system, the sympathetic adrenal, was constantly and irregularly overworked or worked in jerks and spasms; while the other part, the para-sympathetic sedative system, hardly had a chance to function. It was this para-sympathetic system, we realized, which was called into play when we made these slow motion movements with sensory feeling, and it was this system which reported the pleasant feelings to the brain and gave us joy. So from this we developed a totally new form of bodily movement–paraplay, the technique of rhythmic movement in slow motion, as slow as the growth of a plant.

Without going into all the scientific detail, which took many years of study and experiments with hundreds of human beings obtaining these same results, we came to the conclusion that these joyful bodily movements we call paraplays are what the ancient physicians gave to their own children for body suppleness and flexibility. That in the misty layers of time and the mildewed pages of books, these practices have been covered up with metaphysical and esoteric superfluities, and sometimes degenerated in use into strenuous exercises in the West and sensational body contortions in the East, is owing to no lack of sincerity on the part of their teachers, but rather to the great discrepancy between our present detailed knowledge of practical sciences and their actual empirical practice, the difficulties of language translation, and the lack of synthesis of modern science into a coherent science of being.

The synthesis achieved by Pundit Acharya in his correlation of the methods of these early physicians enables us to lift the mists of time and restore this ancient science to its original meaning as a science of *agelessness* leading to individual integration. The methods are simply the *knowhow* of being eternally young in every cell of the glands and organs, bones and tissues of our body. It is not how many years old we are or even how long we live but how fully alive we are at any age–intensely alive in every cell of our body from the edge of our toenails to the top of our head.

G. A. Brooks

YOU HAVEN'T SLEPT

INTRODUCTION TO PART ONE

Owing to the researches of many great scientists, we know what happens during sleep in the blood and the brain. We know that there are special sleep tissues in the brain which secrete an acid called hypnotoxin inducing sleep. It is not this acid condition of the brain called ordinary sleep with which Doctor Acharya deals in this book. Here he is concerned with the fact that unless the brain has at least four hours of *sound sleep*, the brain cells may not get their Nissl granule foodstuff to replenish the energy dissipated during the day's work.

The paraplays of release given in "You Haven't Slept" are intended to take one beyond the acid condition of ordinary sleep into that realm of profound slumber and perfect sleep where one may tap the "reservoir of life" to recharge the batteries of the brain. This secret of hibernation is known to many animals such as the bear in his winter cave and the birds on their tiny perches with their heads under their wings, but somehow this knowledge has been lost to man. Here in this section one may learn how to regain his lost heritage by simple techniques of alkalized relaxation called paraplays of release, bringing into play the para-sympathetic system of nerves to quiet the sympathetic system and sedate the whole body.

Perhaps in this simple reversal of excessive motor activity of the body lies the possibility of arresting the rapidly mounting motor diseases of our age!

NICHOLAS VIGGIANO, M.D.
Piermont, N. Y.

1

A WORD

They have taken complete charge of the tree.

Loud names—these are. They are busy cleaning the tree. Trimming it.

Still louder names are spraying venom fumes over it, to free it from parasites, and even plant lice. They are experts.

They promise flowers and fruits from the tree. Theirs is the red passion . . . these names, who have the tree, branches and leaves and all.

My Maker has made my hands clumsy that I tend only to the roots. My fingers shall only caress the soil, toiling with the fertilizer. My eyes shall remain bent to the lowly, where the seed was.

So, without a voice, I sit on the dust, and wait . . . at the root, I wait . . . .

May it please my Master.

I.

NEED OF SLEEP

"I haven't slept a wink last night!"

How often you have said that. You and you and you.

And you have said it without knowing what you are saying.

When you say you haven't slept a wink, what you mean is that you haven't been satisfied with your sleep, because sleep should give complete rest.

The trouble is you regard loss of consciousness as sleep. You do not know the full significance of sleep. It will be shown in this book that sleep is rest and recuperation of energy rather than unconsciousness.

Let us tell you the most important thing. Sleep is a vital need. Sleep is life. Sleep keeps our longevity and health by an infinite physiological detailed process. Yet sleep is not what you think it is.

In this book we shall tell you what is sleep and how mankind can learn consciously to go to sleep and enjoy sound sleep.

First of all, let us tell you that sleep is more necessary than food. We say sleep is more necessary than food, because without proper sleep you do not digest your food. Without proper sleep you suffer from bad elimination, that is, constipation; and without proper sleep you are irritable all day long. Your nerves are on edge. You worry. You fret.

Without proper sleep you blame circumstances. You plan things wrongly. Without proper sleep you cannot make money. You cannot meet situations as they come up.

Without proper sleep, you make your life a chaos. You fall victim to therapy after therapy, drugs, quackery, psychology and what not.

You would be surprised to know how many of your misfortunes and failures are due to improper sleep. Furthermore, you would be surprised to know that people in high places, educated and otherwise, have seldom known real sleep. They, too, are the victims of situations similar to those which have confronted you.

You cannot understand this wholly, because human nature (meaning the human body) *compels* the whole body and the mind (meaning the brain) to go to sleep in spite of one's mind. This profound and proper sleep without man's being conscious of it, is the thing that keeps him going. God and nature keep him alive in spite of himself (meaning his mind), but he knows nothing about it.

In this century man shall consciously taste and experience the sweet sensation of sleep. Would he learn the meaning of sleep, he shall know that the body and the brain material are like *batteries which become recharged with the infinite energy from the atomic world around him, as well as from the food atoms in his bloodstream and the electrolytes in the protoplasm of his body.*

This recharging has got to be complete for a complete man. A fully recharging body and brain with the nerves plunges into the magnetic fields of this earth and once more stirs up all the solar energy outside and inside the body.

Let us get along with the story.

II.

SLEEP EXPLAINED

Sleep is half of life, the most important half. In saying that sleep is the most important part of life, we are not being poetic. We are scientific.

Sleep takes you to the only and true reservoir of life.

So that it becomes perfectly plain we say to you, *as though* there are two of you in you. That is, you the body, and you the mind. Now when we say you the body, we do not mean you the kind of body we see in the mirror. We only mean your internal organs that keep up your life process and the circulatory system, the process of digestion of food and elimination of it, and the unceasing oxidation.

As against this body, there is another you which you call yourself, meaning your mind: your consciousness.

We are separating your internal organic being from your mind, so that you will understand thoroughly and practically what we mean by sleep and your needs of sleep.

Of course it is understood that there is no real difference between the brain and the body because the whole thing is one.

We repeat, sleep takes you back from your mind to the reservoir of life itself to be recharged with the life energy. Please read this carefully as science demands minute attention.

Life energy is stored up in the protoplasm of the cells of the body in the form of electrolytes. Your sugars, calcium, sodium, sulphur, magnesium, iron, phosphorus, etc., etc. are always present in the protoplasm in the cells of the body. When their supply is diminished, they pick it up from the food you eat, which is carried by the blood through the corpuscles themselves.

This never-ending source of supply to the cells of the body by the circulation, and the cleaning up of garbage and end-products of the body by the same circulation, goes on perpetually by the action of the visceral organs—the heart, lungs, stomach, intestines, colon, kidneys, etc.—and also by the help of glands which whip them into action.

Now all these vital life processes, meaning this incessant supply of energy and life, go on outside of the mind and consciousness. Your mind or consciousness, which is the recordings of the brain cells, is not responsible for, nor can it directly and permanently interfere with the vital life process.

We want you to understand this once and for all, that your mind (your consciousness and thoughts: the workings of the higher brain cells known as cerebral cortex), is not in control; nor can it control the process of the gathering of food by the cells from the food that you take in through your mouth. Your mind can interrupt and interfere and degrade this process to a large extent through the sympathetic nerves as agents of the brain, but it can never stop or degrade it enough so that the body would be permanently hindered.

Furthermore, mind or the cerebral cortex with its consciousness and thoughts gets its food and energy from the great reservoir of the body.

Consciousness the Beggar Mind

Your consciousness and thoughts, that is, the cerebral cortex, the mind that helps you to think and feel and control the voluntary muscles of the body—all day long, during the entire waking time that you are conscious and thinking and thinking—this mind merely spends out and wastes the energy supplied by the body, dissipating it to "smoke," meaning gases and end-products.

Mind retains very little of this reservoir of energy for itself. In fact, the beggar mind (consciousness and thoughts: meaning the cerebral cortex) has to beg its own energy food from the body itself, food which comes to the brain by way of the bloodstream.

All the mind can control is the voluntary muscles. Remember

this. It is very important that you understand this fact, especially you, the *mind over matter* therapeuticians.

Now this process of food gathering and food distribution, known as metabolism of the body, which goes on with the blood circulation and the workings of the viscera—heart, lungs, etc.— all of which are giving food to the cells and also doing the cleaning of the body, is like another human being outside of your mind. Thank God for it.

Now that you fully understand the two of you in you, you must once and for all know that this heart, this liver, lungs, spleen, kidneys, intestines, colon, all these organs and glands are not under the control of your cerebral cortex or mind; for they are under the control of your midbrain, which is at the end of your spine at the base of your brain.

Midbrain Is Independent of Mind

Midbrain does not think. It is not conscious, or subconscious or co-conscious or anything of conscious. When people say "Nature cures," they are referring to this midbrain. This brain is autonomous or independent of your consciousness—the mind or cerebral cortex.

For the layman, it is sufficient to understand it is as if there are two brains. One is where the consciousness is, or the topbrain. The other, toward the head where the spine ends and the topbrain begins, is the midbrain which has no consciousness.

Now the incessant, never-ending, ceaseless work of the heart, lungs, stomach, intestines, colon, kidneys, circulation, etc., etc., which are working and working and working without stop until a person dies, is under the control of the midbrain.

The upper brain of your mind is only a *waster*. It can only jump with pain and pleasure coming *from the body through the nerves to the brain*, but it cannot create one iota of happiness, nor can it manufacture any food material or energy for the life of the individual.

Now read carefully what we say. After reading, study it and understand it for all your lifetime—because it is sacred to us and nothing is more important to you than this knowledge.

The Reservoir of Life

Sleep takes you from your mind, the cerebral cortex, to the realm of this domain of the midbrain, that is, the domain of the body and the visceral organs.

When you go to sleep, you, meaning not your consciousness, but you the life, put the upper brain or cerebrum to sleep, and you become real life in the realm of the organic self, meaning the throbbing protoplasm of the body itself.

Now you understand what we mean by the *reservoir of life.* We mean this ocean of food and energy material where energy is bubbling in the storehouse of the protoplasm.

A perfect return to this reservoir of life is perfect sleep—better known as hibernation.

There are perfect Yogis who have trained their being to give their body energy to the brain (meaning mind), and their brains are eternally calm as floating on the surface of sleep. This is something you will not know without ages of practice.

But what you shall have here will be a perfect rest, sleep or   ˙
hibernation, for six or eight hours a night, so that you will be able to enjoy perfect health, free from the attacks of the sympathetic nerves—free from the poisoning effects which the blood and the kidneys cannot eliminate fast enough.

God knows the average person of the twentieth century has not known sleep. He is more or less—it is only a question of degree—suffering from nerve poisoning. In the sections entitled "Breath Is Life" and "This Precious Heart," we have continually pointed out, with every pugnacious thought or pugnacious impulse and disappointed thought of the brain, the brain cells and the nerve cells continually give out "skunk juice" and poison.

The only time one can get rid of this poison perfectly is in a state of perfect hibernation or perfect sleep, as we shall show.

If you will not get alarmed and can understand the real meaning, we shall say that sleep is merely a preparation for death. We will not explain that in this book because you would be scared and think we are preaching annihilation. It will be sufficient for you to know that we are giving an injection of real life and rejuvenation.

Whether you are a workman, a clerk, a salesman, a great executive, a soldier or a sailor in the armed forces, or merely an ordinary citizen of any geography, you will find here the secret of vital life.

You must learn what is sleep and how to sleep, so that when you wake up in the morning, you become and feel a younger creature every day.

Sleep is bathing in the life energy.

The ocean of life energy is in the protoplasm of the body. The beautiful rise and flow of the current of life is going on perpetually in the body outside of the consciousness and mind of the individual. Here is the real you.

The question is, how you shall learn to dip your cerebral cortex and mind into this fathomless depth of the reservoir of life.

Here we shall give you exercises which will get your mind by the neck and keep you down in the depthless hibernation for a few hours every night. That will be learning how to sleep. You will get the result the very first week. You cannot fail to get results, even though you might be the last word in education with a string of degrees from a university.

Now turn the pages and go on with the story.

III.

MECHANISM OF SLEEP

So that you will fully understand the mechanism of sleep, we draw this picture for you.

Let us understand that your cerebral cortex or mind is a powerhouse generating electricity, sending out currents, mostly to the voluntary muscles of the body. That means your arms, your legs, your face muscles, your nose, throat and eye muscles, etc., all those that you can move, turn, twist and control.

Now this electrical energy of that part of your brain called your mind, is continually using up the electrical material (meaning electrolytes) from the powerhouse; and as it is sending the current through the nerves, making the voluntary muscles work, it is also making the voluntary muscle cells use up their electrical energy.

Compare this with the federal government, which is taxing the populace but is not concerned with the minute detail of the local government, which is under the control or direction of the village, county or state. Understand that in this two government system, they act as independent partners although ruling the same individual.

We are speaking of the federal government, which is a luxury compared with the local government, which is a primitive one and fundamental.

The Spendthrift Brain

Now this brain government, this brain powerhouse, is not concerned so much with where its own power material comes from. It is continually busy in spending and spending and spending out its own energy of the brain, and also the energy of the voluntary muscles by making them work.

The most of the time, when this brain or mind is awake and you are quietly sitting down, it is thinking. You, the mind, are sitting down and thinking. This thinking means the mind is using at least the eyeballs, and indirectly but very effectually straining the heart and the lungs by the onslaught of its electrical wire agents, known as sympathetic nerves, through the respiration of the lungs, the heartbeat of the heart, and an occasional spasm of the stomach.

Understand this generating station, this electrical powerhouse known as brain, your mind. This brain is connected with a system of pathways or electric wires, called the sympathetic system. Every time it is aroused, meaning the brain is excited and emotional, it begins to work on the muscles through the nerves. It begins to interfere with the digestive processes through the sympathetic nerves. It begins to make the heart beat faster by the sympathetic nerves. It begins to make the stomach juices, intestinal juices, pancreatic juice, liver juice, and the saliva juice of the mouth dry up by acting through the sympathetic nerves. Now these nerves are the electric wires coming from the brain, or your mind, outside to the voluntary muscles, and inside to every part of your body, everywhere.

You begin to understand the cerebral system or mental system. This is "hell on earth." This system wastes energy but does not create energy. You cannot be a fit citizen of the twentieth century unless you understand that, whether you are ignorant or educated, you are a victim of this system.

This cerebral system will ruin you, unless consciously you learn to free yourself from it. This secondary powerhouse continually not only spends energy, but damnably interferes with the very creation of energy in the body.

Body Protoplasm the Reservoir

Now against this wasting type of a powerhouse, thank God, we have a reservoir of energy, a fundamental powerhouse, and that is the electrical material of the powerhouse remaining in the *cells of the bones of the body*, in the *cells of the muscles and tissues of the body*, in the *walls of the blood vessels* of the body and in the *muscles* of the internal organs.

These cells generate body electricity. They themselves co-ordinate among themselves and set up a government, a central station with a local president known as the midbrain. They have an electrical wire system of their own, that is, the nerves known as the para-sympathetic system. These organs, muscles, bones and blood create energy and store up energy. They have come from the days of the seas. They have come from the plant, invertebrate and vertebrate kingdoms until they have become the body of man. These cells have counted ages and ages of history. These electrolytes in these cells are elemental. You could easily see there is an ocean of energy in their protoplasm. If they are conscious, they are divinely conscious with this universe in a way which mind will never know. They give us a sense of well-being and good health.

That's where the Being is. In the electrolytes of these body cells.

This vast potential mass of energy, electrical and electronic in its nature, is continually floating in this universal energy of the solar system.

These cells of the body get their foodstuff or electrical material not only from the food that comes through the mouth and becomes vitamins; but these cells get their food from the rays of the sun, and oxygen from the air by ingestion. They get their atomic food from the water we bathe in. The cell protoplasm gets its minerals when we sit on the soil or handle the soil with our hands. They thrive and work well in empty space. They enjoy the gloom. They are in tune with the universal rhythm which they have learned from the seas, that is, to rise and fall.

Now you understand the work and rest of the lungs, of the stomach, of the heart, of the intestines and all your other vital organs. Their rhythm is the rise and fall of the seas.

These organs never overeat. The doctor may give all the oxygen from the oxygen tank, but they will not take any more than they need. The mind can give all the devitalized and poisonous food through the mouth that false appetites and advertisements may devise, but the stomach, the intestines, the colon and the kidneys will try to get rid of it.

These body cells have the experience of ages and ages and ages through evolution. The mind of man or cerebrum cannot corrupt them. Fundamentally they remain unmodified.

Therein lies our heredity–that man shall last forever so long as this earth lasts. After that, they (these cells) will go to another atomic world. You cannot destroy them. They will always remain in this universe in one form or another.

Now you understand this limitless and fathomless and ceaseless energy of this most powerful generating station. This is the body we speak of.

Sleep, therefore, is the process by which you come from the mental station to this motherhood of energy.

Oh, God, how long will opium and opiates help you to come to this reservoir of energy! What Coney Island psychology can ever teach you to come to this fathomless bosom of energy? What can mind do or learn by words, words, words?

Learn to come away from your mind to your real self, the organism.

In this book on sleep we are sowing the germs of a gigantic philosophy, where the twentieth century human being will learn to come from the cerebral self to the organic self, so that a greater human being will be born thereof.

You learn to tell your mind right now that it is inside of you and not outside. You are beginning to see it is not "mind over matter" but gigantic matter teaching and sustaining the baby mind.

The man who wrote *Man Unknown* was looking for a cerebral man because he had never looked for the real man. He had never tasted life in its fathomless being.

May God express himself in your sleep.

IV.

DESPERATE NEED OF SLEEP
AS ENERGY SOURCE

In view of what we have learned in the previous chapter, we begin to see that the brain material with its agents, the nerves, continually needs from the body the supply of energy that comes through the bloodstream. Brain or mind needs the energy food which is called carbohydrate, as well as oxygen.

It will be shown that the carbon and oxygen, the exchange of these two gases, called oxidation, carries on the electrical energy. What is left over from the energy are carbon dioxide and other end-products, which we call garbage and which the blood cleanses from the brain and takes to the lungs to get rid of it.

Now you pay attention to what we say and remember this all through your life. This exchange of the two gases, carbon dioxide and oxygen, is the life process. It is called oxidation. Whenever oxidation takes place, the result is two-thirds heat and one-third action.

When you are thinking in that brain, then oxidation is taking place. That is how you think. Therefore, the more you think, the more is the heat in the brain; the more you worry, the more is the heat in the brain; and the more emotional you get, the more is the heat in the brain.

Then there is another way your brain gets heated.

Light is made up of rays, so is sound. The light rays from the outside world, as well as the chaotic sounds from the outside world, are pouring into your brain and continually pricking the brain cells to work. And overwork in the brain means overheat.

A machine called an electrometer has been invented by which they can actually measure and show us the electrical curves of the storms in your brain. What these neurologists do not tell you emphatically is, that during these storms when you are thinking hard, worrying, or being emotional, etc., the inside of your brain is steaming hot.

At these moments and hours the rate of flow of blood in the brain is tremendous and terrific. The blood is bringing food supplies, such as carbohydrates and oxygen to the brain, and the brain cells are eating them up, using them so fast that it is beyond the imagination. You could easily see how on such moments the body is deprived of food.

How Energy Is Wasted

On these moments when your brain is excited, your heart, lungs, stomach and intestines, all the parts of the body that manufacture energy, are terrorized. Like whipped dogs they are intensely watching what the master brain is going to do next.

The eyeballs and eye nerves, like the reins of a horse, are jerked to and fro, hither and thither during your emotional moments. Your poor lungs are spasmodically taking in oxygen and giving up carbon dioxide by exhalation in spasms and sobs.

During this time, several parts of the voluntary muscles, either the arms or intercostal muscles, or some other parts, are terrifically tense. In other words, these muscles are burning up their sugar energy.

All this process, therefore, which the civilized creature calls thinking, is a process of mere waste of energy.

Then, not only that, the most of the time he is "gabbing." Talk, talk, talk. Oceans of words coming out of his mouth. The speech center in the brain, the word center in the brain, and most of the parts of the upper brain where mental pictures are photographed, are kept working terrifically, wasting this energy and creating heat.

The scientist measured this body heat by a unit of measurement called calorie. How many calories of this heat are dissipated by this thinking process, do you think?

We shall call all this energy—Nerve Energy.

You will see in the office buildings, in the universities, in the streets or wherever civilized people have gathered together, you will see they have gathered to waste this energy. You could easily see what has happened to the smooth circulation of their bodies when they are mentally active.

I would like to see a big house with its intricate plumbing system work, if used as the circulating system of civilized man's body is being used. The house will not have plumbing very long, and certainly other parts of the house could never get water if the water is held in one part so long.

There are something like sixty-three thousand miles of human pipes—arteries, veins, vessels, etc.—through which the blood is going, to give food to the body and to clean away the garbage. The greatest tyrant, the brain, so long as the individual is awake, is using this blood spasmodically and creating heat in its own sphere.

This is somewhat of the picture I can give you, the layman, in your thinking, worrying, and emotional moments. This is what you call you. You are going on, on this nerve energy, spending it and wasting it every moment of the time you are awake.

I did not create mankind and I did not make man civilized. I am only a reporter, who, in reporting the inside of man to man, is showing his inside picture to himself. The tendency of civilization is for every individual to be brilliant. How well they can "gab." How they can shine in the eyes of the other fellow! This scattered brain is marching on, thinking, talking, writing and spelling words, words, oceans of words, one syllable of which seldom, if ever, produces energy or brings peace and happiness to mankind.

The question is, do you not think that you need real sleep to replenish this energy that you can waste all day long? Do you not think you need a complete freedom from this brain and nerves for six or eight hours a night *when they will go through* the uninterrupted metabolic processes?

You fill up the stomach early in the morning with a heavy breakfast, then you go to work. The blood that is necessary in the stomach and pancreatic region to digest this bellyfull of food is called up from other parts of the body to do thinking, while working to keep up the smooth process of digestion and elimination. The two vital processes of life, digestion and elimination as well as oxidation, are interrupted by the thoughts and mind of man.

No one can change man. It will take centuries before he will change his habits. All we could show him, therefore, is how to replenish this energy from the reservoir of energy while he is asleep, so the poor thing has something to spend.

Body, the Rich Man

Brain or mind, the rich man's spoiled heir, must have something to spend. Body, the rich man, can give it, if the spoiled brat, brain or mind, with its satellites, the sympathetic nerves, would leave the body alone awhile for six or eight hours a day to manufacture and give the energy uninterrupted.

I hope you are getting a little idea of what sleep is and why you need it desperately.

Sleep is not the grand theatrical performance of going to a silken bed and snoring for a while. Sleep is complete anesthesia of the brain. In this book we are showing you how to learn to attain it.

Please don't be brilliant with this book and read it mentally, then cast it aside. We are giving you the fruit from the tree of life. He who will take a bite and eat, will get a little more of life and happiness. The one who will brilliantly read it and brilliantly say to himself he has understood it and known it all the while, or who brilliantly will cast this book aside and spit on it, will fall victim to drugs, therapies, psychiatry, fortune telling and what not, and join the fossils of the earth to fertilize the ground upon which will be born a saner and safer humanity.

Such is my prayer.

V.

NATURE'S GREATEST GIFT—SLEEP

When you are dangerously ill, meaning when your very life is in danger through infection or other causes, your body doesn't trust your brain. Brain becomes unconscious in this almost state of hibernation. The white corpuscles of the blood, increased by the new juices manufactured by the body while the brain rests, help to fight the germs and the disease; and as soon as the body gets proper food, it manufactures and generates tissues by cell division.

At that time when you are dangerously ill you cannot abuse the body by alcohol, cigarettes, idiotic excitement, or by the brilliant ideas of your brain. The body creates a hush of death and silence of the brain. Colors do not appeal. Entertainment does not appeal. You do not read books, newspapers, or listen to the radio.

If you are to survive the life and death illness, the body at last revolts against your mind and nerves, and hushes them, while *life regenerates life by manufacturing new energy from the protoplasm of the cells* of the body. New tissue cells and blood cells are born.

Quiet, quiet, quiet is all that is necessary. Now, who is this quiet for? The brain, or the body? The brain, of course, is the answer. The one great worry of the doctor at that time is how to keep the blessed brain quiet, so that the nourishment can go through the metabolic process, and the patient be recovered through regeneration by cell division.

This is what you mean by "Nature cures." This is what the doctor is after. That is the crux of the science of medicine. The doctor cannot give you life, but he will make the greatest effort to stop your mind wasting life, what life is creating again out of life material. His one prayer is how to keep your brain hushed.

The soldiers in the army will have soldiers' heart either through enlargement of the heart or arteries. The war workers will have war workers' heart due to the nervous strain and due to the nervous energy expenditure. The average citizen in any walk of life will have "heart trouble" meaning straining of the nerves affecting the heart and high blood pressure. See the section "This Precious Heart" where we show the heart has no trouble of its own, only that *caused by the nerves.*

We shall commit a crime against humanity and against these millions of toiling and sacrificing human beings if we do not tell them the need of sleep and teach them how to attain profound sleep.

You are getting a glimpse of what we mean by sleep: hibernation, an absolute hush of the brain.

We have to show you every little item that excites the brain during your sleep. We have to show you how you will create new habits of life so that you will learn to keep sleep the sacred, vital, all important thing in life.

You will learn, not to attain this sleep by any drug or alcohol, or again by artificial stupor, but how to fall asleep and remain asleep while the body is recuperating, as a healthy child does happily. The next morning you will have quiet nerves, a lot of body energy, and fresh energy bubbling in your brain. Your eyes and eye nerves will be clear as you walk in the air.

Our greatest trouble would be: you would say, "He is talking about the other fellow. I am healthy enough, eat good, sleep well, am very active physically and mentally all day long. I am as strong as an ox. I have plenty of energy, therefore he is not talking about me."

No, we are talking about you. You are using up your nerve energy and your brain energy. Fortunately, through heredity, you have a beefy body and a lot of foodstuff stored up in the protoplasm of your cells. All your brilliancy is nerve material. Your energy is not coming from this organism, nor from the reservoir. In spite of you, your body is luckily supplying the amount of energy needed for the day, during sleep, and also through the unconscious process all day long.

You are not responsible for your good health or sense of well-being. You are very lucky, that God (and Nature in you) is giving you this energy. Now, why not learn to come back to this source of energy *knowingly* and flow along with it? Why continually use the muscle energy by the whip of your nerves?

It is such people who will not get anything out of this book. They are satisfied to suffer when suffering comes. Meanwhile, like a drunken sailor, they will go on spending.

We are talking about you, tomorrow and tomorrow and tomorrow. We are talking about your life and health and real happiness. This can come from the silence of death alone for –

Silence is the voice of God.

VI.

BIOLOGICAL SLEEP

Sleep is not a psychology but a biological process. In other words, sleep is not merely loss of consciousness but sleep is that which takes the organic being known as man, to the reservoir known as his biological self, for replenishment of energy in the flow of life. Only the *truly* educated ones will understand this chapter.

To explain this fully, we have to embark upon a seeming departure from the subject matter, sleep.

We have three kinds of smiles.

Cerebral Smile

When you see the stupid signs in every office building everywhere "Keep on smiling," they are referring to cerebral or mental smiling. By ideas they are trying hard to smile and for half a minute they smile—until the smile fades out into the gloom and worry and the nervous fears of the day.

Man cannot keep on smiling by ideas.

This "salesman's smile" can only create fatigue of the brain. Yet this is the only type of smile man seems to understand. A very noted metaphysician student of mine was taught the organic smile. He enjoyed the benefit of the teaching during his illness. When he got well, he wrote a pamphlet and distributed it among tens of thousands of his following telling them to "keep on smiling" as smiling will cure all physical and mental ailments.

Biologically he himself got the benefit of the organic smile but he preached the cerebral smile to his following. It shows how hard it is for an intelligent man to understand his being. Cerebral or mental smile is a social affair. Man's love affair is only cortex deep. His pleasantness and spiritual thoughts and whatever he designs as pretty are only skull deep.

Let this be the lesson of the age: *Man cannot smile mentally.*

Thalamus Smile

The physiologists, next, speak of a thalamus smile.

At the base of the cerebrum, that is, the lower part of it, is the ancient brain. Here are the thalami. These thalami are supposed to be the seat of the bodily emotions. The thalamus smile is a sense of well-being *felt* by the body. When the body is giving this sense of well-being to the thalamus, the thalamus reports it to the mind. This thalamus smile is a sort of a feeling of well-being that every healthy and young being of a man or woman can feel without any self effort. Mental effort seems to hinder it by the interference of the sympathetic adrenal system.

In another volume we shall explain these smiles at length.

It will be sufficient to get on with this story here and show the real smile of the *being* in this chapter.

Organic Smile – Amiya

The nerves of the whole body, as well as the brain with their endings, continually secrete either honey or venom juices.

Whenever the organism is threatened as to its very life, it secretes a venom secretion. As the stink stone. As the stinkweed. As the bedbug. Or as the skunk. In the section entitled "Breath Is Life" we have pointed out that these juices come out of bodily fear.

In utter (and mind you, we have no other word in English but utter) safety, the body, meaning the organism, feels really happy. And the nerves of the body, meaning the para-sympathetic nerves, with the help of the vegetative system, secrete honeyed juices: chemical secretions which are conducive to the flow of life and happiness.

When this honeyed secretion I call *Amiya* is present in all parts of the body in the nerve secretions, all the glands of the body secrete the necessary juices also. The bile flows well, the enzymes of the stomach are happily active, the pancreas is giving its insulin. Such a person does not need any insulin shot from a doctor. Even the reproductive glands become filled with juices. The being feels as though the entire vessel is full.

The circulation and vasodilation bring a flow of radiance over the surface of the whole body.

The eyes of the animal dilate and become soft and happy.

The breathing is soft and easy. Even the odor of the mouth of such a creature is like the perfume of a flower.

The thalamus sense of the outside world and the body temperature is cool and soothing.

The organism feels the lightness of a feather, as though all his flight and bird instinct are revived once more.

This is the *organic* smile through the honeyed secretions from the nerve endings of the body. This smile can only come from *perfect ionization between the cells and the neurons.*

That man could live seven hundred years can be understood from this standpoint. Such a man becomes theoretical because mass consciousness degenerates his biotic being by the cerebral process.

We are speaking about something very important and very useful this day to every worker all over the world and particularly to the soldiers in the army and war workers.

Man has only learned to punish his flesh and exert his muscles by the whip of the brain and mental ideas. Physiologically speaking, the pyramidal tract of the central nervous system jerks the muscles to spasms, drunk with the adrenal juice of the sympathetic adrenal system. The result is fatty chemistry of the muscles. Farther result is strain of the sympathetic nerves to create overheated conditions in the brain. The final result is jerky on the heart so that at the end of the day and at the end of the war, the soldiers and war workers have soldiers' and war workers' heart to the joy of the cardiographists and digitalis makers.

How much of the coronary trouble of the heart, how much of the thickening of the arteries, how much of the high blood pressure in old age is due to this pyramidal tract tyranny of the muscles, and sympathetic nerve tyranny of the vegetative organs, has not been fully studied by the physiologist.

Now, suppose the worker learned to *feel* his body – the body juices and bodily smile first through training; and now, suppose he learned to bring all his energy *from* his body *to* the mind in a *flow*. What a tremendous amount of strength he would have to exert without straining his heart and without suffering from vaso-constriction!

Here is an experimental process of bio-physiology of the being. Here is a fulfilled life process. Here we speak of the man who has not stepped out from the path of organic evolution into cerebral degeneracy.

To make it very clear, we charge that mankind so far has been a cerebral and mental creature standing out from his being. As soon as we say *being*, like my metaphysician student, he at once creates a cerebral smile and creates an imaginative being in himself, super-imposed on himself. The colleges and universities have started from the cerebrum and come down to the body. The whole science of mental therapies is based upon cerebral treatment. All gymnasiums and trainings of men have proceeded from this cerebral standpoint.

But the cerebrum is only the twigs, the end of the tree. Life remains at the root and the trunk of the tree. The sap of the tree and all the mineral substances and the water that the root of the tree will give to the trunk, so that beautiful leaves and flowers will be born thereof, have been forgotten. When they say that "God is in you," *Father forgive them, they do not know what they say.* This cerebral creature lives by the twigs and tries to secrete juices from the twigs to the tree.

We catch man in the twentieth century as an abnormal cerebral and mental creature whose consciousness has been divorced from the pulsating river of life.

Our holy job is to hold him by the neck of his mind and plunge him back into this river which is the throbbing universe and solar system.

His body, like the tree and everything else in the solar system can get nutrition directly from nature through the roots. It does anyhow. How much more nutrition he can get from the earth, dirt, plants, the vegetation, the sunshine, the waters, the air and vast space!

His organic self can get these and plunder them so that his body can smile, but his cerebrum and his sympathetic adrenal system do not permit him to do so. As against this cerebral man, the next century will know the *organic man* with a finer and more sensitive cerebrum. To him, the toys of civilization will be mere toys. To this man of mind over body and mind over matter, it is hard to show the organic realm.

The trouble with the mental man is that his body is dry. The nerve endings do not secrete enough honeyed juices. By continual tyranny of his vaso-motor system, he chokes his glands and organs, and his body is filled with nerve poisonings. He is dry. He is sharp and breakable. He is like a piece of log that is all bark. He is all brain and no pure healthy body.

The twentieth century man or woman is an eating, sleeping, walking corpse. In one word he is dry.

The job is to wet him with the live juices.

The task is to teach him to go back and fall in the river of life practically.

No amount of preaching and scolding him will help him until we show him the organic river and show him how to throw himself headlong into this river. The trouble would be, he will still try to plunge into this river cerebrally or mentally. It cannot be done.

Our continual experiment with hundreds of students at our Institute and elsewhere has shown us that some of them are too far gone to understand the fountain of life.

It is especially hard to show this man organic life when so many cerebral institutions of quackery call his attention. He only understands muscle training by the mind. Or he understands vitamins and drugs from the outside world, either from a bottle or pillbox. The task is to hold him by the neck and bring him back to his organic self.

Sleep is the beginning of that process. This sleep is therefore not ordinary sleep.

One may easily understand then, what we mean by sleep is to

take him to the other side of the river. Sleep shall teach him to cross man's world, man's consciousness: consciousness of things, to the blind, deaf, soundless, rayless, depthless fount of protoplasmic life.

In the brain there is a will center. We do not mean the volitional centers of cerebral effort. The difference between will and volition is, will is of short wavelength and requires no effort. It is an effortless effort. It is an inclination to give up effort. It's an effort where all motor impulse and action cease. It is a dissolution of the mind. It is the last and utter surrender of the conscious electrical potential.

We need *this* instrument of will to teach him sleep and life.

VII.

THE PRE-REQUISITES TO SLEEP

If the layman cannot remember or understand anything in this book, he will at least gain great help if he will read this chapter carefully and remember what is being said here.

In the first place, there is an ignorance and a world propaganda as to the hours of sleep.

One must definitely understand, it is not the hours but the *quality* of sleep that is the need of the individual.

Sleep to the layman for all intended purposes should be like anesthesia to the brain. A complete death of consciousness for at least three hours a night.

Here are eight conditions absolutely necessary to sound quality of sleep.

1. Pitch darkness. A place where not a ray of light is permitted.

2. A hush of sound where not a ray of sound is permitted.

3. A cool breezy place. Where the temperature is very pleasant, neither hot nor cold, and where a very, very gentle breeze is stirring.

4. No peripheral disturbance of the body by the creases of the bed sheet, or by any other touch of anything that might wake up the brain. What is true of touch is true of smell or odor. There should be no obnoxious odor or perfume or sweet smelling flower in the room, however delicate it might be.

5. A half-empty stomach. That is, the stomach should not be empty or too full, so that a lot of undigested food in the stomach will create dreams.

6. A very pleasant state of mind before going to sleep. A pleasant state where the mind will not be full of plans or worry. A complete mental curtain of the last act should be rung down before going to sleep. Everyone should go to sleep with a blissful prayer for the happiness of the world.

7. A receptivity on the part of the nerves of the brain must be dropped by the will. This will be explained later.

8. Laziness is a detriment to sleep.

1. Pitch Darkness

If you go to sleep in a place where there is light of any sort, you will not sleep soundly. The light rays can penetrate the eyelids of your eyes and poke the brain to work. So long as the optic nerve, the retinal nerves, the visual purple process or the optic thalami of the brain would be excited by even one ray of light, the brain, meaning the cerebral cortex of the mind, will keep on working.

"Petit" perceptions will go on in the realm of the brain. What ordinarily the psychologists call subconscious, is actually the irritation of the brain. Distorted ideas will go on in the brain. These disturbances will not permit complete hibernation of the body which is the aim of sleep. The sympathetic nerves by the vasomotor process will keep on disturbing the vegetative organs of heart, lungs, intestines, etc., also the pituitary, thyroid, adrenal glands, and even the liver and pancreatic glands.

The least disturbance of the brain will be a complete disturbance of the organism.

Complete death of light is therefore necessary to sleep.

The man or woman sleeping in any room with any kind of light does not sleep. No wonder they dream!

2. Hush of Sound

What is true of light is true of sound. One ray of sound would

be just as bad as a ray of light. We have found that lightlessness
and soundlessness alone are sufficient to quiet down the nerves
and soothe the brain.

Quite a few years ago, I took several nervous students to the
Endless Cave near Harrisonburg, Virginia. After five minutes' stay
in this vault of darkness, where there is no light or sound, the
students felt as though they had received a new lease of life, their
nerves were so soothed.

In blind cases, as well as in many nervous cases, where our
students practice Samadhi, we have found that it is the light and
sound rays which are the real cause of the nerve troubles and brain
confusion.

Neurological investigators in New York, Germany, France and
England have found that sharp noises cause lesions in the brain.
We have gathered the data of all these neurologists from all
different quarters of the globe. They show that sharp noises like
the crashing of the subways cause spasms of the stomach. These
neurologists have also found that a room full of women
"gabbing" equals a noise similar to the noisiest part of Niagara
Falls, amounting to one hundred decibels of noise, the highest
register of noise. These noises not only hurt the brain, but through
the vaso-motor system, cause spasms in the heart and the vital
internal organs.

Noiselessness, therefore, is an absolute need to sleep.

3. Balance of Heat and Cold

There is a wrong idea among human beings all the world over
that we continually need fresh air. People open up the windows at
the least suggestion and talk about getting some fresh air in the
room. What people suffer from, when they are crying for fresh air,
is not lack of fresh air, but stuffiness. It is a question of the
temperature of the room or the moisture of the room. In almost
every livable room there is always enough oxygen present. Air is
not pumped out of the room. All air contains about two-thirds

nitrogen and one-third oxygen. Now there is plenty of oxygen in
the air present in the room. When anyone says, there is not
enough fresh air in the room, what he means is, the room is too
hot.

Life is a perfect balance between hot and cold. Plainly speaking,
life is a balance between the heat inside the body and the heat
outside touching the surface of the body. The solar system keeps
up this balance of heat for the vegetable and animal kingdom. The
slightest variation from this perfect balance is a threat to life.

Overheating a room causes discomfort to the whole organism
and particularly to the breathing. Overheat in the brain causes
unhappiness.

Some day neuro-physiologists instead of psychologists and
psychiatrists will find out that the lack of happiness of man is
merely an overheated condition of the brain and a carbon dioxide
gas preponderance in the brain.

It is sufficient for the laymen to know that an overheated room,
and overheated brain will keep his nerves and brain boiling, and he
will not go to sleep.

What is true of heat is true of cold. In an extremely cold room
or even slightly cold room, the circulation will fight to equalize
the heat balance between the body heat and outside heat. During
this fight, the nerves in the brain will keep on fighting. And the
person cannot rest.

Therefore, the absolutely necessary condition to sleep is a cool
room where an invisible, imperceptible, soft, gentle breeze is
stirring. A fan would be a detriment and stir up the air, as the fan
would mean noise and the fan would give spasms of air.
Remember, we emphasize a cool room and not a cold room nor an
overheated room. An overheated room lowers the vitality by
lowering the metabolism.

Too much heat is an enemy to man. Too little heat lowers his
life. Fat women take heat therapy. This lowers their vitality by
lowering the metabolism which is so necessary to reduce their fat.
Ignorance is responsible for it. We emphasize so much about heat
and cold because the average person has not known real sleep on
account of sound, light and the wrong temperature of the room.

4. No Peripheral Disturbance

No disturbances of the body must take place during sleep.

You must not sleep with anybody. Not even with a cat or dog. You go to bed to sleep and not for socialization. Let all socialization end at the edge of the bed. The bed should be a canoe to take you to the other side of the river.

If there are creases even in your bedsheet that touch your toe, it will wake up your brain without your consciousness or knowledge.

A soft bed or a hard bed is merely a stupid propaganda. There should be a high pillow (not too high) to rush the blood down from the head, because you do not want too much blood in the brain.

The kind of bed the body will feel most comfortable and relaxed in, is *your* bed. The bed must be spacious. The bed must not have heavy covering to put too much weight on the body. Do not carry a load when sleeping. The least bedclothes the better, providing you do not feel cold.

Finally, we remind you that anything which will touch your body in the slightest degree will start the local reflexes, and if the stimulus is strong enough, it will poke your brain and you will have disturbed sleep.

Remember, one ray of light, one ray of sound, the slightest deviation in temperature, the slightest touch of the skin, can wake up the brain.

5. A Half Empty Stomach

There is a propaganda all over the world that you must take something hot in your stomach to help you go to sleep. What the whole idea amounts to is this: heat the abdominal region and draw the blood there, so the head will feel empty and fall asleep. What a stupid idea! In half an hour or so, the metabolic process as well as the material dissipation of heat will undo this method.

If you eat too much and the stomach is loaded, this extra work on the overloaded stomach will create a disturbance inside and give peripheral disturbance to the brain.

We said a little while ago that nothing should touch your body. The inside of your body is like the outside. Any gas condition in the abdominal region will cause disturbance to the sensory nerves and wake up your brain. The gas condition practically pokes with a bayonet and disturbs the brain. The stomach should be half empty, just working mildly so that it does not wake up the brain.

The stomach should not be completely empty either, because if it is empty, it will have the pangs of hunger, which is merely a sensation from the stomach region through the sensory nerves to wake up the brain. Some light digestible food must be left in the stomach to work upon, so that it does not get hungry. Understand, hunger is merely a need of the stomach and not always a need of the body. An empty stomach will keep on disturbing the brain.

We shall not go into the subject of digestion, nutrition and elimination here. It is sufficient to point out that a heavy meal like that of your dinner takes from seven to eight hours to digest. The stomach gives out a little bit at a time, by opening the trapdoor with the help of the hydrochloric acid, to the intestines to digest. The stomach is a storage place of the food you eat for seven or eight hours. Therefore, go to sleep at least four hours after this heavy meal after at least half of this digestion has taken place. Do not reload the stomach then with anything more before going to sleep.

If you have formed the habit of eating some supper an hour or so before going to bed, this habit will create a sensation of hunger in the nerves of the stomach. If you satisfy this old habit, you will keep your brain awake. Change that habit of the spoiled animal called stomach. You are the master and not your stomach.

6. Ringing Down the Curtain

Do not go to sleep in the arms of society. Do not plan, worry and think of serious things before going to bed. Here we have to change the lifelong habits. In one second drop the mind, the brain, to a fathomless pit of darkness and noiselessness, and sense of nothingness—and with one smile go to sleep. Our exercise for this will be given subsequently in this book.

Do not keep on thinking what he said and what she said, however sweet their sweet nothings may be. Are you going to sleep or celebrate? You had better keep awake if your day's celebration is not over. If you must worry, get out of the bed and cool your brain.

Here the other conditions to sleep will help you a lot. Here our exercises will teach you how to sleep. In sleep you are going to be your other personality, your organic you. The knowledge of the human species with their things, things, things, must die now completely. Sleep is a bath. It must cleanse your brain. It must recharge your batteries.

Sleep like death demands that the knowledge of the human species die out completely during the short period of three or four hours. Heaven knows you have plenty of time to celebrate the human consciousness during the waking hours of the day.

In one word, sleep is the *death of human language.* Words, even the memory of words must die out in the brain. *Here* is the supreme secret.

A touch on the skin will wake up your brain. Gases in the stomach will wake up your brain. Inside the brain itself, the flicker of an idea will wake up the brain. One mental picture of sight, sound, smell or any sense of stimulus, just the same as from the outside world, will wake up your brain and disturb sleep. A complete collapse of brain vitality is required so far as your consciousness is concerned.

The brain should be left without an effort. To effortless effort.

7. Curtain on the Brain

Sleep is a complete change from one world to another which I call *crossing the river.*

Here we must say most emphatically that one has to train his will to give up volition. It is hard to explain this to a layman.

Therefore, without being technical, we shall explain it this way:

What man calls his waking life is nothing but a series of sensations coming from the outside world to his brain, and a series of sensations going on, from the brain pathways to the body. This inclination or desire on the part of the brain to receive sensations from the body must be dropped in a split second. Here the brain must learn for the first time in its life to drop sensations in a split second and melt away into a smile. This is the birth of the will. All the neurons of the nerve cells that receive sensations will thus get a dose of opium. The brain and body will at once secrete a secretion.

There is a small bunch of tissues at the base of the brain called sleep tissues. They secrete an acid called hypnotoxin. Its fumes permeate the brain and cause sleep. It is a definite chemistry.

In the same brain also there is a will center in the frontal lobe. Will is in inverse ratio, diametrically opposite to volition or brain effort. What the average person calls consciousness is brain effort. Will is directly and diametrically opposite to mind.

Will starts by pulling down the curtain on the brain or mind. *Will dissolves* all human effort.

Birth of will is a delicate training by the supreme neurologists known as Raja Yogis.

The training of the will is the job of a century. It is the most difficult job. What man suffers from is degrees of disease of the will (Abulia). The neurologists cope with it in its abnormal form. The permanent cure of neurosis cannot take place until the will is born. No drug or chemistry is known to give birth to will because the *will is a generation of a tremendous voltage of the brain.*

The will center works when all other centers of the brain are absolutely senseless and inert. Will comes in such a fraction of a second that man's consciousness cannot perceive it. We can only observe its function. As soon as will appears, the entire brain as well as all the nerves seem to give up their receptivity. They receive no more sensation. The body and mind seem to emerge in a delightful bliss where there is no more human consciousness.

Through our years of experiment with thousands of people, we find that the average person has glimpses of this will in spite of himself. We have also found that the average person, without the help of any drug or chemistry, can train himself to train his will.

In another book dealing with this phase of neuro-electronics we shall deal with will at length.

Here the layman will be given the opportunity and the training by an exercise which will teach him how to generate his will and kill all receptivity in a split second. We insist it is a training and a life practice.

Do it and you will live happily. Don't do it and you will live unhappily the short life you live.

8. Lazy Body Cannot Sleep

Lazy people do not sleep well. Laziness is particles of sleep. When the body is lazy, it is a partial hibernation with a mild toxic condition. A lazy person cannot go to sleep because he or she has been sleeping all day long in waking hours. You can easily understand a half-burned damp piece of wood cannot burn well and cannot give fire. For the layman, it is sufficient to know that he must work physically to earn sleep.

Laziness must be defined. A lazy person could do tidbits of physical work and consider himself to be overworked all day long, but in between laziness has never wakened up the body completely during the day.

Therefore such a lazy body has not a very good circulation all over the body during the day. Such a body has not used up the food material that came in or which is present there. Such a lazy body has not eliminated and excreted well. Therefore, the recharging of "half-baked" batteries is difficult.

One must work physically all parts of the body by sitting down, getting up, walking and standing, and especially bending the waistline, if one wants to sleep well at night. A woman can go like a top all day long window-shopping and "freeing the world" in social clubs and public gatherings, yet her body has not worked uniformly.

Body is a protoplasmic mass. Every part of this protoplasm must work, inside and out. Swimming is an example of this work. Mountain climbing is another example. The best example of work is tree-climbing.

We are not prescribing this climbing or swimming every day. In our work of body oxidation, we are pointing out that man must repeat the last of his vertebrate and invertebrate stages of existence, to live fully without pounding his heart by the jerks of his nerves.

An exercise will be given in this book for real work, where the abdominal and the pelvic regions would really work.

We have found the secret. We have found that old age, senility, disappointment, sickness, lethargy–the most of these are due to heavy buttocks. When a man or woman gives up all the life energy to beefiness–to his or her buttocks in the process of sitting down and keeping on sitting, either day-dreaming or doing office work– the body has become thoroughly lazy.

Giving up to the buttocks is old age, causing bad elimination, constipation and bad circulation. And the shortest time reaction to lift the buttocks from the seat is youth and regeneration. It is the pull of the buttocks without pumping the heart that is the real work.

When the invertebrate was becoming vertebrate and developing the pelvic region and the buttocks, it wriggled this part of the anatomy. In mankind this part of the anatomy has gradually become set.

You could easily see in swimming, in mountain or tree climbing, in sitting down on the floor and getting up from the floor without the help of the hands, how this part would be exercised. When you have done this, you will begin to understand what we mean by physical work and what we mean by laziness.

Please do not jump to conclusions, and start to work this part without learning how to work it without punishing the heart, or you will have what they are beginning to call a "soldier's heart." You will be given this definite exercise of doing real physical work as violently as a steel worker or a soldier has to do it, yet without hurting the heart. It is so easy when you learn the physiological trick.

Here it is sufficient to know that lazy people will not sleep. Laziness means laziness of the back of the body and not the front. Laziness is laziness of the spine of the back. Laziness is laziness of the pelvic region and the buttocks. Even miles of walking would be laziness. Even an all day's work by a housewife would be laziness, because while walking in doing the household work, she has not bent the body and has not exercised that important part of the anatomy where the hinges are. The lower abdomen has some very vital organs. The upper abdomen has the solar plexus, the brain of the body. These are the parts that must work to have real work of the body.

Without this type of work a person will be regarded as lazy. And lazy people will not sleep.

VIII.

FREEDOM FROM HUMANINGS

We assert that the average brain (and all of our brains are average), does not get enough rest either awake or asleep, to recharge itself for the next day's work. This would be very difficult to prove unless the student is willing to experiment on himself and understand the meaning we suggest thereby.

There are three types of consciousness in the average brain.

1. The Occupational Consciousness

He or she not only works at the occupation, but the most of the time talks and thinks about it far more than works at it. Yes, even long after working hours, the brain is a cauldron, a boiling pot of these ideas of the occupation. Yes, that goes even for a college professor of the most brilliant mind in a high place or in the artistic world. Even a metaphysician who prays for thousands and gives advice to thousands, may become a nervous wreck every so often therefrom.

2. Socialization Consciousness

When the brain is not boiling and brewing the occupational consciousness, it is busy with what he or she or they have said or have left unsaid or should have said or should not have said, etc. This socialization consciousness includes hopes and disappointments, ambitious planning and fears, health and illness, remorse and reverses, etc., etc.

Mind you, this consciousness (as most of the consciousnesses of the brain) has "I," "Mine" and "Me" for a center, around which are boiling and flitting around to boil all other human beings—all the world in fact.

3. Window–Wishing Consciousness

There is another type of consciousness that comes in the brain due to any happenings to the sense perceptions. I shall call this window-wishing and window-shopping consciousness. That is, any stimulus that comes to the eyes, ears, touch, smell, taste, the brain responds to it and holds on to it like a bulldog to a stick. Until the next stimulus comes.

Of course, this is a part of the socialization consciousness also. In fact, the classification of these consciousnesses is artificial and meant merely to help grasp the subject.

The story is that the brain boils with ideas of human society. And the story is, that the average person goes to sleep, that is, when he has to go to sleep, in the arms of the human society. Therefore, even in his sleep, all parts of the brain do not sleep.

Experiment with sleep has shown that the average person does not sleep soundly more than two or three hours at the most, and that even is interrupted sleep. The best way to experiment with sleep is to observe the breathing of the sleeping person. You will notice that in sleep, the breathing does not remain shallow, light and regular. Personally, I haven't found two dozen regular respirations in a person awake or asleep, except in some of our students when they are practicing Samadhi (hibernation).

Now, neurologists have found brain lesions caused by sharp noises, glaring flints of light and other physical shocks to the periphery. Drugs, nicotines, alcohols, and accidents can cause brain injury. Some day a great neurologist shall find ultramicroscopic injuries in the brain due to words, words, words, the human language. In this book, however, we are dealing with a practical problem.

These millions of workers who are working in the factories and shops, the millions of white collar workers, and these thousands of important executives, including the "brain trusters," must be taught *brain rest*, or freedom from continuous and unending human thought processes.

That they cannot sleep well is partly due to this habit of the brain boiling. Psychologically, the "I," "I," "I" consciousness is the process which we shall call *Humanings*. There is a way to get out of it partially for the sake of brain rest. Without this new habit of the brain rest, no one would know the sweetness of a sound sleep.

Here is the prescription. Please set aside one tiny hour out of twenty-four hours a day, faithfully. During this hour, go where there is no artificial light, preferably in utter gloom. Or go and practically, physically touch with your hands and as much of the body as possible, dirt, earth, grass, vegetation, plants, and water in the midst of Nature. Go in the snow. Go in the sunshine if possible.

Now this is the most important part of the prescription. Please go *alone* and do not take your *Humanings* with you.

Associate with plant, vegetation, dirt, earth, water, air, space, gloom and the white light of the sun. Stretch your whole body and being with yawnings and pour yourself, your whole bodily self, by continually yawning with your whole body, into the stream of Nature.

Stay away from friends for one hour a day. Stay away from the thought of human beings for one hour a day.

There is the reservoir of protoplasmic life. The protoplasm is crying for space, air, sunshine, gloom, the earth, dirt, the mineral substances, vegetation—plants and trees, and water, water, water, water—and rocks and mounts.

Steal away from your human society and yourself, from your friends and relatives and your own social mind, and give yourself up to the living God. Go to the fathomless, endless detail of the solar system *materially, physically,* and practically, and not mentally.

And not mentally.

Keep the social mind, *Humanings*, behind for one hour a day. Your poor eyes would rest. Your poor nerves would be soothed, the heat of your brain would cool. Please, please, please go back to your mother in her motherhood.

This prescription we are giving is vital to man, workman and brainy man alike.

For a merely meager one hour a day, please try to be alone. Free from books, newspapers, magazines, radios, moving pictures, parties, cigarettes, alcohol, noise, music, gabbing, thinking, and all other stimuli of the mind.

Some day you shall die. And there would be a complete hush of your senses. Be bold and face this stark reality and you will be a better man or woman. Life does not come from vitamin pills, radio programs and newspaper headlines. Learn to create the habit of going back to life for at least one hour a day. Learn to get complete silence and hush of your senses in the human realm.

I am not wasting space and your time of reading when I say, please pay attention to the following few lines.

Please do not go to Nature to do any favor to Nature. That is, do not try to bring the human consciousness to the plants, to the gloom, to space, to air, to water, but learn to commune with them by *dissolving* into them. Let *them* speak to you—to your brilliant mind. Let them hush you one hour a day and *give* you their vitamins.

You are a tired brain child. Let your real mother soothe your tired eyes and tired nerves and tired mind. Let her, with her gentle hands soothe your fevered brain at least one hour a day, so that you will sleep well and will have restoration of energy for tomorrow's work.

I know it is very difficult to teach human beings to go back to the source of energy, because of their mental habits. You understand opium habits, alcohol habits, cigarette habits. You know the insistence of these habits. By continual therapy, one can change these habits. But the worst and most harmful of all habits is the mental habit we call *Humanings*:

Human habits of Nerve Pathways in the Brain. The psychologists call them concepts. God knows, that God alone can change these neural paths. Therefore, we plead with you to go back to the living God to become a part of Him for at least one hour a day.

We do not know your language—meaning thereby, we do not know any words which will not arouse argument. Words will not give you the essence of the request we are making of you. But, somehow, we know you'll understand.

We are pleading for your health and your rest. We are pleading that you will learn to go back to the reservoir of life. Please do not argue with words in the maze of words. We have used words as a vehicle through which we are trying to appeal to your heart.

In the heart of your hearts you understand profound, depthless, manless rest. Therefore, create the habit of going back to the fathomless joys of silent Nature that is only vocal in beauty and not vocal with human soul.

This is a precondition to sound sleep, the real rest.

Meanwhile for you we pray in silence.

IX.

SLEEP FOR THE BRAIN

We are not dealing with the superficial matter of common sleep.

Our task is so difficult because we have to convince the educated people of the world that mankind needs a newer education about the body and the brain.

Medical students in whose hand the health of nations has been placed, are the ones whom we should approach beseechingly. Our appeal to them shall be that they should study this subject matter sympathetically.

Medical students, while they study how to take care of man in their different classes of study, generally pay real attention to anatomy, physiological materia-medica and internal medicine.

Lately they have been studying a superficial science called psychology. When they study the central nervous system, they regard the nerves as merely electrical wires to carry messages to and from the brain.

When these students attend the classes in biology, they pay more attention to the details than to the whole. Morphology, true bacteriology – the whole subject matter of biology is studied from the standpoint of therapeutics, rather than a thorough understanding of the organism as a whole.

It is not because their professors in the biological classes do not explain the whole of the organism. It is not because their professors do not continually pound on their head that the cell is a living matter and can take care of itself if the brain and the nerves do not interfere with it, but the medical students do not pay very much attention to that. The average medical student depends upon therapeutics, drugs and psychiatry. He forgets the heredity of the protoplasmic masses. He forgets that the cerebrum is the last spoiled child of the organism. He forgets that the cerebrum merely celebrates the joys and pains of the organism but has no joy or pain sensation of its own.

The student forgets that the visual images in the cortex continually whip the association center of the brain and keep the oxidation and the heat going. He forgets that the ideational processes of the brain continually interfere with the vital knot in the medulla oblongata, and by sending pressor impulses to the heart, keep the heart in jerky movements and in "hot water" all day long.

He forgets that with the least ideational stimulus in the brain called consciousness, the motor impulses poke at the respiratory center of the medulla oblongata and make the phrenic nerve jump and the diaphragm jump so the respiration becomes chaotic. He forgets that the vaso-motor system, controlled by the ideational processes of the brain, keeps the vegetative system and the glands starved and choked and dry.

He only pays attention to the blood sugar, the wrong functioning of the liver and bile, the overloaded kidneys and too much secretion of adrenal glands, due to the nerves from the brain. But he forgets that he is continually told that the organism with its vegetative system can generate its own insulin by its pancreas if the poor pancreatic glands are left alone by the sympathetic adrenal system.

What the student forgets is that the brain, brain, brain, the cerebral cortex, through its vaso-motor system causes continual vaso-motor constriction and wrong vaso-motor dilation, and thus plays havoc with the poor animals of the body: the vegetative system and the glands.

Desperately he tries to make use of his psychology and psychiatry, and desperately he relies on ampules to retrain his thyroids, his adrenal and pituitary glands, his liver and his pancreas, and so on.

He forgets, for billions and billions of years, these animals have come through all difficulties and have withstood the onslaught of insurmountable difficulties of nature. They know what to do in regard to the organism. They know that they can regenerate and keep up the process of vitus, the life, if they are left alone by the nerves. The circulatory system can go on smoothly just by the laws of osmosis and dialysis, and by the laws of bio-chemistry, if the cerebral cortex would only leave it alone and would not interfere with the vaso-motor agents.

We say all this because *Cerebral* people are at the helm of nations. Because people who love ideas rule and teach mankind – people who are sick themselves.

It is the holy duty of a new education to teach mankind to come back to the *protoplasmic* realm of the organism from neck down. Here man should replenish his energy to soothe and quiet the cerebrum, so the cerebrum can be cool and be a bigger brain in the future.

Today man's brain is overheated. The rate of flow of blood in his brain is continually causing storms. Endocephalographic showings are in vain. Psychology cannot train his brain, his neural habits. And the tragedy is, the more brilliant he is, the more he will use his brain and cause tyranny to his eye nerves, respiration and heart.

Students of medicine, who are real students of biology, will at once understand what we are driving at. Here is a life and death struggle between the cerebrum and his central nervous system on the one hand, and the massive protoplasm known as the body with his vegetative system known as glands and circulation on the other.

The heredity of the organism wanted to give real nutrition and health to the central nervous system and the cerebrum, so that the frontal lobe of man's brain could generate such ultra-violet and other rays of shortest wave lengths as to contact the heart of matter. Wasteful and spoiled child, the cerebrum, through the nerves, would not do its own work but debauches itself in the sensations of the peripheries, and thereby punishes the peripheries by the vaso-motor system.

The job of this age is to teach the brain to keep it drowned in the protoplasmic mass of the organism.

Ampules or vitamins will not teach the brain. It will not teach new neural habits. Evironment, meaning newspapers, books, radios, discussions, studies in the universities and what not, the end-products of the human cerebrum can only create chaos of stimuli for the cerebrum itself.

'Tis too late in the day of the process of evolution to stop these phases of man's civilization.

The best way to make a better man of him is not to tell him what is the matter with him, but teach him the practical, positive method by which he will get results and be a better man. We have to train him by changing his entire polarity. Today he is living from the brain to the body. Tomorrow we have to teach him to live from the body to the brain.

The body protoplasmic mass must hold the reins of the nerves in the cerebrum. Sleep is the beginning of it. The kind of sleep we refer to, therefore, has to be a drowning of the brain and the nerves in the fathomless depth of the body ions.

We assure you, our experiments have shown us that in a few weeks it relieves high blood pressure, heart trouble, neurosis, bad digestion, bad elimination, strained eye nerves, and so on. Why not? Does not the cell of the body know what to do?

Does not the body cell regenerate? Even the neural axons and dendrites? What prevents them from so doing? The vaso-motor system. The sympathetic adrenal system.

We are not writing a medical book. Therefore, we hope from these leaves, the students of medicine will understand what we mean by sleep. By sleep we mean hibernation. By sleep, we mean the brain going back to the body for further energy to waste.

You could easily see all the war-workers and millions of white collar workers would be efficient. They would live longer. They would not have enlargement of the heart if they shall have learned how to resign to fathomless sleep—at least a few hours a night.

Will not the doctors teach them this? Will not the science of medicine pay attention to the science of biology? Will not the science of medicine take away its eye from ampules and vitamins and psychiatry and look back to the oceans of ions composing the organism with all its unbeatable heredity and unmodifiable instruction!

Somehow we know man is about to turn back from "mind over matter" to the matter over mind. *"Thy Will be done,"* meaning the universe will speak to his brain.

How long shall we poke his brain with drugs and psychology to repair the patchwork of injuries in his system? Will not his medical advisor teach the average man that his own body is the real medicine? He became man by the protoplasmic struggle through ontogeny and phylogeny. From his conception to this day he became man by the cell struggle. Do not the cells know how to struggle? Do not the cells have the plant heredity and animal heredity, meaning invertebrate and vertebrate? Do not the cells have the heredity of the jellyfish to the highest vertebrate? Do not the nerves from the brain cripple them?

Sleep will teach man without his consciousness how to be rebaptized by the flow of life and the honeyed juices of life.

One need not worry about being lazy if he has learned perfect sleep. One ray of light or sound is enough to wake up the brain. Modern civilization, the environment is nothing but light and sound rays. The cerebrum will never remain asleep. Only man's brain will learn to be cool, a little more sane and less nervous – more coordinated.

For his health and happiness we mutely pray.

X.

BIOLOGICAL EXERCISE

One of the greatest causes of disturbed sleep, let us call it "ill sleep," is constipation. Gases generated by the putrid matter in the intestines disturb the sensory nerves. The nerves carry the sensation to the brain. Thus parts of the brain alternately keep awake. The sensations are weak, and therefore they do not wake up consciousness.

Nevertheless, "petit perceptions" of the incoming sensations from the abdominal region keep portions of the brain busy. So in the darkest, most noiseless, and cool room—in the most comfortable bed—a well satisfied person cannot sleep well because of constipation.

We do not understand constipation. Unless one suffers pain or great discomfort, one thinks one is free from constipation.

Let us think of a coal furnace. It is the oxygen in the air that makes the coal burn. A million dollar a pound coal will not burn well unless the furnace is cleaned out of every speck of ashes. The heat you get out of the furnace is equal to no ashes and free passage of air.

With the human body clean, the small and large intestines will keep healthy. Any food you eat must be *fully*, completely and absolutely digested, and the residue cleaned out. Now, who is the furnace man of the human body?

Please pay attention to the most important thing in your life. We do not care how educated you are, please pay attention to the *meaning* of what we say. The average reader reads alphabets. Please read what we say and get the point. It is your life and death.

The furnace man to clean your garbage is the *Intestines* and not you or your brilliant mind.

Intestines are involuntary muscles. Your mind over matter can only cause pressure near the anus, and strain the heart and the back of the neck, but cannot touch the intestines to eject garbage.

Civilized people drug the intestines to eject garbage. The only thing they know is drugging. Advertisements of laxatives and purgatives go on and on. The manufacturers and their families, as well as those who prescribe them, are victims of these drugs. Lately, the vitamin fans are trying to drug them in a new way.

They forget that it is not the million dollar a pound coal that is important in a furnace. The furnace man who will clean the ashes is the most important agent. In the human body it is the intestines themselves which must work.

You see, since man's mind cannot *poke* the intestines directly through voluntary pressure, he lets drugs (including vitamins) do it for the mind. Do you get the picture? Do you understand? You can "lead the horse to water but you cannot make him drink." Scientists are discovering new pokers and becoming famous. They are amassing fortunes. Yet they, too, are victims of constipation.

We cannot argue with you. You who would say you are not constipated. We cannot show your inside to you and show you how you are gathering garbage. Unless and until your mind registers pain and discomfort through gas and at last sick kidneys, we cannot show you your inside. The fact is, you are always constipated—more or less.

The greatest message of the twentieth century to mankind is that man's intestines are causing constipation. Therefore his brain is also constipated. He is unhappy. Man's brain is seldom cool and seldom has the perfect carbon dioxide balance. The greatest cause is abdominal constipation.

Please do not laugh it off.

Here is the remedy.

The remedy does not come from man but God. Therefore it is very simple. All simple things, God's things, Nature's things, are very hard for man. His complex mind will kill him. If he wants to live and progress, be really educated, let him cast away his vanity, his garb of the university degrees, and humbly come back to God. We are not preaching religion but biology.

Intestines are live animals. They are autonomous. Man's mind cannot touch them. Thank God, man's mind cannot move them.

Animal intestines have their biological habits of taking food from the stomach, digesting nutrition from whatever food they get through the mouth, and rejecting the garbage. Ceaselessly, without rest, all the time they are working. Cells of the intestines are taking turns at eating and resting, and working, working, working. Bad food, which is drugs, meaning chemistry, is hurting them. Yet they are working. They have learned this work from their very organic existence, call it God.

Now something ungodly has happened in modern man.

The species man was preceded by the quadrupeds. Man's arms and legs are really heir to the quadrupeds' four legs. The quadrupeds use the hind legs in such a way that one leg takes a forward move and then the other leg does the same, alternating. As it moves then, it moves its behind from side to side. In so doing, the four-legged animal moves all the bones, muscles, ligaments of its behind, the leg bones, pelvis, etc., and thereby, also through nerve connections, continually moves the inside of the abdomen and the intestine. Here, the intestines with all other organs worked concertedly, practically.

Then came the tree climbing biped using its behind bones, muscle, pelvis more strongly. The stomach and intestines were greatly stirred up.

Then came the gradual biological and organic downfall of man.

The primitive man at least climbed trees and irregular mounds and mountains. Up to the horticultural and even agricultural age (before he began sitting on a tractor, etc.), the uncivilized man sat on the ground and got up from the ground. He, at least, used his legs irregularly, thus causing motion of his intestines.

This the modern man, against his God, wants to do by taking vitamins Q, R, S, T, Z. The false health messiahs want to cut off the biological lineage of God and Nature and make man an artificial, technocratical, chemical, vitaminical creature.

This son of Adam and Eve is ashamed of his animal heredity and wants to forget it. It is too bad he has a *sinful* body–he wants to be all brain and control the sinful intestines by mind over matter. His God, his spirit and his soul are in his brain, to wit head, and not in his vulgar, indecent intestines.

But now, the vulgar, filthy intestines are eating up, swamping the God in his brain.

How un-Godly is this man! He sits in a chair in a university classroom and hands out concentrated wisdom to his guild while the chair breaks his back. All his degrees do not touch his intestines! He learns biology, the theory of evolution from books and writes books of biology, and the biological creatures, even the cats, die laughing looking at his spine and pelvic region. He cannot even bend. He will crack to sit on the floor.

The exercises therefore are given only to remind man what he organically is—how to be normal, meaning organic. To re-establish his heritage, his lineage with the biological tree.

Walking with a stick or a poodle dog is not exercise. Prize fighting or baseball playing is not exercise. Abdominal twisting in a beauty parlor is not exercise. Muscle swelling with dumbbells or gymnastics in a gymnasium is not exercise.

All such exercises take you toward death instead of life by causing "athlete's heart," "soldier's heart," and many other abnormal heart conditions.

In concluding this chapter, we have to perform a difficult duty. Ill sleep and ill health of modern people are due to three bad things they take through their mouth. Moneyed barons, manufacturers, would like to tear our flesh for recording this. But we are at "our Father's business."

1. Bad food, that is, food from which we get no nutrition.
2. Cigarettes.
3. Alcohol.

One more thing that we take through our ears—
4. Noise (subways, trucks, radios).

One more thing we take through our nose—
5. Foul air of the cities.

Another thing we take through our skin—
6. Overheat from our apartments.

Two more things that we do not take through our skin—
7. Sunshine in the open air.
8. Free water of rivers and seas.

And the greatest crime we commit against our own body —
9. Sitting on a chair and not sitting on the ground —
   on the soil, and handling soil and vegetation.

God help His man by bringing him back down on his feet.

XI.

EXERCISES EXPLAINED

The exercises we are giving you are paraplays of release: a new type of exercise totally different from all others which are gymnastic or muscular. They are going toward *effortless* effort bringing into play the para-sympathetic system of nerves.

These exercises will create new habits. Practice them often until you have formed new *physiological* habits.

In insomnia, high blood pressure and heart trouble, they are inimitable.

Never do them quickly, sharply, violently, or strenuously.

As you take these exercises, do them slowly, languorously, flowingly, so you get sensual, *pleasant* sensations. Only by being slow will you have graduated motion without jerks or creases.

The first series we are giving you will teach you how you can master sleep at will. This is the first thing you do in going toward—

Perfect Sleep—Rest for the Brain

Exercise i
Release the Jaw

1.

Sit in an easy armchair.

2.

Start mouth breathing. Open your mouth slightly and drop your jaw. From now on, do not breathe through the nose.

It matters very little whether you breathe hard, deep, or soft and low. In a few minutes your breathing will tend to become regular and shallow.

Nature will so adjust itself that it will automatically cut out the "gas" supply. You will not take in as much air; therefore, the oxidation of your body as well as brain will slow down. Automatically your muscular actions will be sluggish and slow down.

This mouth breathing alone will be the first step toward sleep.

Exercise ii
Release Internal Smile

1.

Now, while you are softly and gently breathing out, you start to smile internally. Keep on smiling inside your body and not with your lips and face. (This is called thalamus smile as against cerebral smile or the social smile of a salesman.)

Your nervous habit will start your brain or mind boiling: meaning, you'll begin to think and thus forget to breathe through the mouth and smile.

2.

So force yourself to come back and stay in this state of mouth breathing and smiling.

Exercise iii
Release the Neck

1.

While sitting in the easy armchair, now begin to slump the head and upper part of the body a little.

This will quiet down your breathing and heartbeat.

2.

While in this state, infinitely slowly, with almost imperceptible movement, "break" the back of your neck. Feel as though you are losing all control of your neck, and let the head slowly fall on all sides, alternately . . . slowly and slowly until you feel your head is becoming empty. You know how an infant has no control over his neck. You become this infant and lose the control of your neck, especially the back of your neck.

3.

Keep on that mouth breathing and smiling. As soon as tension and tightness return, go back to this state.

Here you will see your impatience will start to disturb the whole thing by thinking, but as soon as you come back to the start—

4.

Drop all thoughts and smile internally.

Your trouble will be you will mentally watch your sensations.

The essence of all these exercises is *feeling* and not watching. Please, please feel these sensations, merge in these sensations, be lost in these sensations and do not watch mentally.

Exercise iv
Release the Joints

1.

Now while slumping in the armchair with mouth open and sagging, and smiling with a "broken" neck, feel that your shoulder and arms from the bone and joint are "broken" and slump these.

In other words, give up your arms from the shoulder blades

completely, and feel as though they are hanging from your body like rags.

2.

Stay like this as long as you can without thinking. As soon as thoughts come, smile more–inside.

Exercise v
Release Pelvic Region

1.

Now feel your back and waistline and pelvic region are also "broken," so that you can't hold the legs any more . . . .
Your neck "broken." Mouth open and sagging.
Arms "broken." Wrist "broken."
Back, waist and pelvis "broken."
Now you feel weak. As you feel after a long illness. You haven't much vitality left. You haven't enough strength to lift any muscle, arms or legs, etc.

2.

Please feel weak like that. Just stay half-smiling.

By the time you are in this state for a few minutes, you are very sleepy. While it has spread inside your body, you shall have found out from your sensation what real rest is. You shall have found a heavenly, soothing feeling is spreading all over your nerves and you loathe to stir up activity in your body.

3.

Just glide along with the sensation and slowly go to bed.

A few times of these five paraplays shall be the greatest teacher to teach you quiet and internal peace, which no drug or sedative or food could ever give you.

Physiologically you will learn, meaning the body itself will teach you how to go to sleep and have a quiet rest in a few minutes' time.

In this type of sleep you are learning the invaluable lesson of hibernation.

The first few times are the hardest because of the nervous impatience of the student. Until the old habits of impatience have been replaced by new habits, the task is difficult. But by the degree the student will taste the "juice" of the sensations of the body, the brain of the student will be bathed in the sensations and will begin to like the sensations, to look for them, seek them, and thus learn how to generate the sensations without very much effort.

The first step of sleep, therefore, is to enter into another world. All day long we live in a world of effort. The door to sleep on the other hand is effortlessness which must be a sensation, a perception, a feeling and never a thought.

We give you the physiological tricks, physical tricks with which you will beat down your mind. We have discovered these with deep and laborious research in the field of nerves within neurology.

The benefits derived from these exercises are so great for general health and rejuvenation that one can hardly estimate them. They must be practiced to be realized.

The trouble with educated people is that they will try to give the dog a bad name and hang it. They will call it hypnosis (which means sleep), and will never realize the sedative possibility of the nerves themselves. They will never understand how the para-sympathetic nerves spread a new juice and fumes through the body with the help of the sleep center (sleep tissues of the brain), and the pituitary, thyroid and adrenal glands.

Only practice will show the result.

What the average person does not know, whether he be a great scientist or just a layman, is that he is continually the victim of eye exhaustion and end-product poisoning of the eye nerves and their fibers.

One may see that he can hardly think without using his eyeballs. He does not know that even in his sleep he is calling upon these nerves of the eyes in his dream process. In other words, the most abused nerves of the whole mechanism are the eye nerves.

All day long practice these simple little paraplays for release of eye strain.

Innate, meaning inside, pitch dark and *absence of all color* is the rest for the eyes. Therefore to go toward—

Perfect Peace—Rest for the Eyes

Exercise i
Release the Eyes

1.

Close your eyes for a few minutes, and keep down your eyeballs. Don't try to look up.

It will be the hardest thing you have ever done in your life. You will notice with every ray of thought, I say, *ray* of thought, the temptation to move the eyeballs upward will come.

2.

Even if it hurts you, try to keep down the eyeballs for five minutes. Let the poor eyes rest.

3.

This will be easier if you smile with your eyes.

With this rest of the eyes, there is a change of chemistry in the brain and the whole body—too deep to study here.

We cannot request you to change your conditions of living and so not strain your eyes. All we could possibly ask therefore is that you release your eyes by smiling with them.

Please understand, rest for the eyes not only implies the food process for the organ of the eye and cleaning of the garbage from the blood vessels of the eyes, but also a continual quieting of the entire brain, therefore a sedation and quieting of the whole body. This is the only way to neutralize poisonings by the end-products of the eye nerves, and secondarily, many other nerves.

You know that by exhalation or spurting out the carbon dioxide from the lungs, you throw out the poison or end-products, and automatically allow fresh air to come. So practice—

Exercise ii
Daily Exhalation

1.
Take a deep breath and blow it out through the nose and the mouth with the sound Ahhh! Do it three or four times.

2.
Do it again, and again, and again.

3.
It is like a duck comes out of water. You understand now what is meant by "water off a duck's back."

Now a student might see that this very moment you are suffering from eye strain. In other words, you have a hard look in your eyes. This moment you have tension of the eye nerves. So relieve the strain by—

Exercise iii
Eye Exhalation

1.
All of a sudden, just like blowing off your breath, just clear out your eyes and *smile* with your eyes.

2.
Break the tension, and bring infinite release. Smile fully with your eyes, and *decrease the intensity* of the sensation.

3.
Keep on smiling with your eyes and make it pale—and pale—and pale until you don't feel the strain of the eyes.

4.

All day long clear out your eyes and soften them—soften your look.

As you inhale deeply and spasmodically during emotion, so you continually excite your eyes spasmodically and deeply during such emotion and through your thoughts. So throw out the end-products. Exhale through your eyes and smile with them. Don't smile with your lips and grin, but—

5.

Smile with your eyes. Feel the soft quality by lessening the intensity.

Smile with your soft eyes.

The best type of eyes is silent eyes, smiling eyes, quiet eyes. These are magnetic and attractive. They show character and inner rest of the brain. They do not show the storm of human ailment.

One more thing, as you walk, as you work, as you go about your daily tasks, keep your lower jaw relaxed and thus breathe easily, lightly, without effort.

We cannot completely make you over with a few exercises given in this book. Regeneration is not possible unless and until you become a willing prisoner of all this physiological and neural guidance and form a complete set of new habits of life.

Some day universities of the world, along with the high schools and grammar schools, will understand this sort of biological training and teach mankind a normal method of living. We are pioneering this inspiration without aid from any rich man or government in the hope that the public with the common sense that God has given them will understand this invaluable service. We bear the Cross alone.

Now we are going to give you a couple of bioplays for constipation and general health as you go toward—

Perfect Grace—Rest for the Nerves

Exercise i
Sit Down on the Floor
without the help of your hands

1.

Slowly, very slowly, with open mouth, begin to kneel down on the floor, bending one knee at a time.

2.

Now that both knees have reached the floor, slowly begin to sit down on one side of your legs on the ground without the help of your hands.

Please do not use your hands. Fold your arms across your breast so that you will not use your hands.

This exercise will be of no value if you use your hands or do it fast.

3.

Now that you are sitting on the floor on one side, get up the same way you came down, coming first to kneeling down on both knees and then slowly getting up on one foot, then the other. Do not use your hands in getting up.

In getting up from the floor to the kneeling position, if you bend your head down to the floor, you will get a better leverage.

Please, please, in getting up, do not fight. If you fight, you will strain your heart.

Keep your mouth open, jaws relaxed, and you will have no fight with your breath or heart.

4.

Practice alternate kneeling on the floor by beginning with the right knee first, then the left; and sitting first to the right side, and then to the left side on the floor.

5.

Keep that vague inner smile all the while.

6.

When you have learned not to use your hands, hang the arms loose while kneeling, and feel the wrist sockets, elbow sockets and shoulder sockets loose as you kneel down. This will help to slow down your motion and bring about the inner smile.

7.

Whether you are fat or thin, do this every day.

If you are very fat, the first few times you will try to sit down, you will thump your buttocks. It has been our experience with hundreds of students that every one of them thumps and falls until they have practiced, practiced, practiced—some of them for months.

We have found even the fattest person can learn to do it gracefully at last. They first complain of their stiffness and general helplessness until they have practiced faithfully and become at last as graceful as a child.

Age has nothing to do with it. We have taken men and women past seventy who have kicked like a mule to do it the first time, and at last through practice have become very graceful and supple. We have found the majority want to give up as soon as they have found it hard the first time.

Our greatest difficulty has been to watch people trying to get up and down like this without fighting with their breath. The teacher has to practically bark at the student and hammer the word slow, slow, *slow*, or the student will fight and strain the heart. Here mouth breathing instead of nose breathing will help a lot.

Now, after you shall have become graceful in sitting down and getting up from the floor like this without the help of the hands, you will take the next exercise.

We mean by graceful that you can get up and sit down on the floor without the help of the hands, *without fighting your breath*. That is how we measure your gracefulness. When you will sit down and get up without the help of the hands without using very

much breath and your breathing is easy, then you are graceful.
Until then, practice, practice at least fifty times a day.

Exercise ii
Sit on the Ground

Now that you have been efficient in sitting down and getting
up from the floor without the help of the hands with ease, go
outdoors somewhere near a river or mount or open field where
the ground is not level.

1.

Now start to sit down the same way without the help of the
hands on uneven ground so that one side of your body will be up
and the other side will be down.

2.

Find as many uneven places as you can and alternately exercise
your pelvic and abdominal region: muscles and bones, ligaments
and tissues this way.
This is the next best thing you could do to climbing trees.

We have not to tell you much about it. You shall learn from
yourself. Our only warning will be, do not strain the heart. Do not
fight. Do it so you get joyful sensations in the body.
This uneven sitting down and getting up from the ground, yes,
vulgar soil, stones and dirt, will help you to relieve constipation as
nothing else will do.

Exercise iii
Walk on all Fours

The next exercise you take will sound silly. However it is very
important.

1.

Right in your room, preferably a large room, close the door so
no one will watch you. Get down on your fore on the floor like a

cat or a dog or a bear, and walk on the floor, gracefully just like a cat.

2.

Walk all around the room on your hands and feet, bringing the right leg up to the left hand and the left leg up to the right hand as you walk.

3.

In this way you will alternately turn and twist your hips, buttocks and pelvis. See to it, as you walk like a cat, that you are churning the lower abdomen by causing a motion there.

Your attention should be to the inside of your lower abdomen.

The whole idea is to exercise the muscles neighborly to the intestines, liver, spleen and kidneys, as you walk on your fore on the floor. You shall have learned from your own sensations how you are stirring up and vitalizing your vital organs.

We have an abdominal brain, the celiac ganglion, commonly called the solar plexus, which is the source of all emotional troubles, including bad digestion and poor elimination. In this new type of exercise, you are vitalizing these animals and they will give you better health.

A healthy body alone can sleep well.

God help you.

XII.

THE VITAL

In all humility we approach the great scholars of human body and mind.

In training of the body and the mind, mankind has been proceeding by the wrong path. Attention has been fixed on muscles. From the kindergarten days to the days of the gymnasium, as well as army training and mental training, man has been proceeding to superimpose systems of painful turning and twisting of his muscles and ligaments. All his physical exercises are muscle exercises with the help of the intercostal muscles.

Here the tyranny of the brain by its agents, the sympathetic nerves, tries to modify the same sympathetic nerves until habits, that is, nerve pathways are formed to make the muscles flexible. In the bargain man develops "athlete's heart," weakened lungs, and an overheated brain. In later days he develops neuritis and even thickening of the arteries due to the strain on his nerves including the eye nerves. The back of his neck gets stiffer and stiffer.

In this little message we cannot point out the intricate physiology, that is, neural involvement implied in such physical exercises. Only an expert neurologist, who has profound biological knowledge and who would study patiently the detail of the neuro-mechanism concerned in these physical exercises, will know the harm one does to oneself by gymnastics.

Every time man takes any type of physical exercise he chokes, holds his breath, or has spasms and upsets his carbon dioxide balance—the perfect carbon dioxide balance which is the criterion of life.

Our criticism of man's frailty is not constructive unless we show him the path. But we are powerless to show him the path because of his existing prejudices.

Hereby we are giving a most important information. Previously we gave this information in our book *A Strange Language*. The book is in the libraries of the world. It earned great praise from leaders in every field. But to our greatest regret and amazement, we found that no one understood the import of the news of the century or how to use it. Everybody passed on the lines with philosophical admiration. So again we give the news now when men can use it if they are directed by expert, trained physiologists.

Here is the fundamental news:

1. Man is a mass of protoplasm. In spite of the differentiation and specialization through grades of evolution into bone cells, muscle cells, tissue cells, vascular cells, neurons, brain cells, etc., he is fundamentally and always will remain *protoplasm*.

2. This protoplasm is fundamentally unmodifiable either by outside drug: food and medicine; or education: cerebral nerve interference.

3. The will to live as well as the electrical potential is not psychic but is dormant in the protoplasm in the electrolytes composing it. (Hashing and rehashing of ions.)

4. Cells have memory. The protoplasm knows how to react and adjust and readjust to stimuli and situations. Color variations up to blushing are the best examples.

5. The cell protoplasm retains the greatest life resistance to the outside onslaught of the cerebrum—mind and its ideas, as well as to the onslaught of food and drugs. Vitamin injections may cause new electrolysis and reionize the protoplasm, but it does not change its evolutionary *character*. Therefore, education is in vain.

All this is not new. But here is the practical application to better man—
6. The protoplasm does not need anything from outside except food. Because, since the plant cell days, it has given birth to cell

mobility in the form of animal organisms. All it needs is outside food. The rest it can adjust to life. Therefore, no education of modification should be inflicted on the protoplasm.

The great news is—
Man should not learn but awaken his cell memory, cell heredity.

Organic Man

As we have said in *A Strange Language*, the organic whole man is still a jellyfish, a fish, a plant and an invertebrate; a vertebrate of the lower type, a mammal, and at last a man.

He still ingests like the trees and the lower invertebrates from the earth, from the grass, from the air, from the sunshine, from the water, from every material environment for his foodstuff, as he does with his alimentary canal when he puts his food in his mouth.

He still eliminates the end-products or the unnecessary garbage of his organism through excretion as the earthworm, as the tree in falling off leaves and bark, and as the higher animal that he is through defecation, urination, perspiration and other methods.

Man in spite of his infinitely delicate differentiation such as eye nerves and ear nerves, still follows the lines of stimulation and exhaustion the same as an ant, an earthworm, a cat or dog, or a tree.

In spite of his attempts at modification and education, all of which amounts to cerebral interference, his protoplasm of the body tries hard to throw off and hardily endure the onslaught of foreign matter from without.

When this protoplasm is inflicted upon by foreign food, foreign education, or foreign nerve tortures by the cerebrum continually, its electrical potential diminishes and the man decays and dies because the enemy is stronger than the vital electrical potential of the protoplasm.

Since the days of the specialization of the nerve cells and the brain cells, which unfortunately continually interfere with the vegetative organs and glands through nerve innervations, the massive organic protoplasm can hardly speak its own mind, and submits to the cerebral mind like a tyrannized whipped dog which must die for the cerebrum and its nerves, generally called mind.

The news of the century is that from now on man would learn to educate his body and mind by awakening the protoplasmic memory of his cells by getting the joyful energy of his electrical potential of the protoplasm of his whole body all together all at once—as in the case of organic yawning and floating and swimming and dancing and other movements—rather than tyrannize his whole being by the central nervous system and especially through the tyranny of new invented drugs, vitamins, and psychological appliances.

Here is a startling example to make our point explicit. We have taken an infantile paralysis case and asked the patient to reawaken the mobile part of his body while keeping his brain half asleep in a lazy drowsy state. In this way through injury current we have brought out the dormant vitality or the electrical potential of the so-called atrophying parts of the body.

The point will be more clear if we notice how the primitive man fights the soft or petrified protoplasm of the civilized man's body. The primitive man is agile while the civilized man is stiff. The former climbs trees such as the coconut tree like a monkey. His ligaments, his muscles, his tissues and naturally all his organs coordinate through cell memory and adjust and readjust the whole organism to the tree. He does not learn agility by the mind or by the central nervous system or the brain, but through his organic memory he becomes the typical invertebrate and the vertebrate all at once—which man is.

Here the man revives his body rather than learns, and we the civilized creatures try to imitate this natural trend of life in the gymnasium. Man is still a fish. Man's body and not his mind revives the fish instincts and impulses of his protoplasm. His para-sympathetic nerves fall in with it. The cerebrum is swamped with the sensations coming from the body to the brain while we learn to swim by the cerebral interference through sympathetic nerves teaching the body how to swim.

The leap of the tiger or any other animal is still dormant in the protoplasm.

Life is a leap—the birth of the electrical potential turning into the kinetic stage. Life, that is youth, is nothing but a spring. This spring cannot come from the mind or the cerebrum to the body. Body generates it. This tendency to spring is always in the protoplasm. We the civilized fools try to learn this spring in the gymnasium and try to teach the children in kindergartens and schools the spring of life by and through his cerebrum and central nervous system.

We the civilized fools give strychnine sulphate to increase the synaptic action of the nerves when the nerve cells are dying to bring about this spring and synaptic action by their natural impulse, which is their nativity.

The courage of the Malayan, of the Arab, of the Gurkar men of India comes from the fount of the protoplasm. We try to artificially create the courage by training the cerebrum with psychological ideas and slogans, which become a superimposition upon the protoplasm, rather than a natural and volcanic eruption of the protoplasm into feelings which would give courage to the brain and the brain show the courage in return. In other words courage comes from the practical *sense of wellbeing of life*, from the total impulse of the protoplasm, while we the university fools try to create this courage by manufacturing it in the association centers of our cerebral cortex and try to diffuse it through the sympathetic nervous system to the muscles, glands and vegetative system, which become so easily tired and finally exhausted through our artificial brain stimulation.

Nerve Cell Training

The layman will gain some knowledge of good health by reading this but he must cooperate with his trained doctor to understand the full significance of the exercises that we are giving in this work.

It is impossible to go into infinite detail of the study of the

central nervous system, that is, the study of the protoplasm of the
nerve cells. We dare not even suggest the capacity of the brain cells
and the nerve cells for fear of being philosophical and academic.
We shall constantly keep both feet on the ground and suggest
practical things which will benefit the public. This is written in all
humility of a research student in the field of precious Yoga.

This is the first scientific attempt to study Yoga in terms of the
central nervous system and human brain. Our objective is purely a
sincere desire to stimulate interest in university circles to study the
subject of Yoga from the medical standpoint and not from the
theological or metaphysical angle of vision.

The Methods of Experiment

For the sake of the layman, we become elementary. Man has two
systems of nerves. The first is called para-sympathetic and the
second sympathetic. The sympathetic nerves with innumerable
fibers falling upon the muscles, tissues, organs, glands, etc., and
present even where the minutest and finest blood vessels are,
usually interfere with general circulation and normal organic
functions. Whenever the sympathetic nerves are working by the
brain control of the man, instantly there is a disturbance of
respiration, heartbeat, and strain on the eyes.

Whenever this sympathetic adrenal system is working, there
would be anxiety in the human brain, a little choking of breath,
tightening of the jaw nerves, and tightening of the arm nerves. It
follows that certain muscles of the body would be tense also.

On the contrary, whenever the body and the brain are enjoying
the *perceptual* sensation of joy, the sympathetic system is almost
feeling the effect of morphine in a most diluted form. In other
words, there would be felt a sense of wellbeing and a general
release.

We can explain this statement better by a practical method.
Follow the method correctly, with infinite patience, and with
minute observation and discrimination.

This is the most delicate and subtle type of a new science. We
cannot understand it or practice it haphazardly, however educated
and intellectual we might be.

All the methods that we are suggesting have been experimented upon with infinite patience and unfailing devotion and
sincerity. No one will ever understand Yoga unless one comes into
this new world of patience, faithfulness and study–although the
applied methods that we are giving could be practiced by any
layman provided he does not theorize and follows our instructions
to the letter.

For instance, when we say *infinite slowness*, we mean *graduated*
slow movements, almost so slow as that of the growth of a plant.
Here slowness is a scientific method and not an attitude of mind.
We do not deal with mind but nerve cells. It is a retraining of the
nerve cells so that they will be fully awakened.

Exercise i

1.

Let the student stand up on his feet.

2.

Let the student slowly and slowly (not infinitely slowly) press
against the ground with his feet and heels and whole body.

3.

Let the student now feel the taste of the sensation of nerve
pressure.

He will discover that this pressure of his feeling is reported to
his brain by sensory nerves as an unpleasant sensation, which his
brain does not like and wants to get rid of.

4.

Now, while he is holding on to this pressure, let the student
infinitely slowly take this pressure away from his feet, heels and
whole body. Infinitely slowly.

5.

As he is relieving himself of this pressure, let the student taste
this sensation of lightness and emptiness and release.

The physiology to watch is his physiognomy and breathing to know by the vaso-constriction and vaso-dilation, the tension and relaxation of the muscle cells, the respiration, and color of the face and skin to observe if the student is really getting the taste of this sensation.

The student should do it time and time again until his brain has definitely formed the liking for this release and emptiness of body.

What we are after is to teach the student the physical experience of nerve pressure and nerve emptiness in more ways than one. He should be questioned to find out whether or not he has definitely *perceived* and then conceived this sensation of infinite lightness.

Exercise ii

1.

Let the student now do this thing quickly.

That is, press against the ground with his feet and heels and whole body very quickly.

2.

Take the pressure away just as quickly.

The physiology would show that as soon as he does this thing quickly, he almost feels choked, that is, he holds his breath when he does it quickly and his breathing is interrupted. Naturally his heart is thumping.

It will be seen that—
(1) there is a certain strain on his eye nerves;
(2) there is an overheated condition in his body when he does this with a jerk and quickly;
(3) his jaw gets tight, his neck gets stiff;
(4) his arms and shoulder blades stiffen and tense;,
(5) there is an overheated condition of his brain.

It should be explained that these are all due to the system of "electric wires" in his body which the brain works upon, tensing all these parts of the body. This is the sympathetic adrenal system.

Exercise iii

1.

Let the student shake his jaw a little bit—as though he has taken the "screws" out of his jaw to feel the release to his jaw nerves.

2.

Now let him take the "screws" out of his shoulders (meaning the arms).

3.

The student will now let go of the stiffness of his neck by relaxing his jaw more.

4.

Above all, the student will not fight his breath or take deep breaths as he is feeling the nerve pressure.

5.

With relaxed jaw, relaxed neck, relaxed arms and shallow breath, the student will now feel the nerve pressure and its release by alternately pressing his feet, heels and body against the ground, and then releasing slowly.

Here the physician has to be very observing and see that the student is learning the evil effects that his tension of the muscles and nerves are causing due to the sympathetic adrenal system.

Please do not psychologize by asking him to smile because he knows only the cerebral smile, which is a social idea and not a feeling of wellbeing.

Warning: If the student does not show patience and liking for this new finding of release from nerve pressure, he certainly is not fit to do any kind of work where tremendous nerve strain and shocks will be his constant nerve food.

Further warning: Before the student is given any kind of severe physical training, he should be given nerve emptiness and nerve release training physiologically.

Speed without Shock

Let us look at the case of an airplane pilot coming down at tremendous speed. At the instant he makes up his mind to come down, he holds his breath, tenses his body—jaws, arms, legs by the sciatic nerve—and is suffering from an excited heart and tremendous heated condition of his body due to his sudden and violent metabolic fight. Here is the onslaught of the sympathetic adrenal system.

Suppose he shall have learned how to feel the sense of release in his central nervous system without fighting the breath and by keeping the mouth open and jaw nerves relaxed. Here he is not accepting the shock.

In other words, the receptor nerve cells are not giving the sensation to the cerebrum, so the cerebrum does not wake up the association centers of memory of fear, but falls into a para-sympathetic joy of the sense of play—as the pilot is about to plunge his airplane in the flight.

Whatever we might put in writing, the expert physiologist will find it difficult to grasp the full significance of these exercises unless we study these things together with infinite detail and observation. This science is new, so new that any preconceived idea will eclipse the meaning of all our findings.

Flexibility without Strain

The physical training of the average man has been in the past, as also at present, in terms of muscle training. We have paid very little attention to the effect on the ligaments, nerves, respiration and heart. We have also paid very little attention to the overheating of the brain.

The future man shall be trained physiologically and not muscularly.

Somehow or other we have studied man as a flesh and blood creature. Study of physiology will emphasize this fact to mankind that he is a nerve creature. Muscles are flexible but for nerves and ligaments. It is the joints that get stiff and are set. Every time we try to make them flexible by turning and twisting, we do it with tremendous fight with the respiration and heart and increased rate of flow of blood. We bring about interruption of general circulation of the vasomotor system because we put the emphasis on the muscle objective rather than the nerve objective to be gained.

Laws cannot give physiological training. It is the job of practical neurologists who understand the sympathetic adrenal system and nerve secretions with their ever-varying ionization with concomitant circulation and effect on the vasomotor system to show to the skilled teachers, health officers, and all those in charge of public health, that they are dealing with neurological creatures and not flesh and blood creatures as such when they are dealing with man.

This will become more and more apparent as we begin to take these exercises with joy and a sense of play rather than learning new tricks.

Exercise iv

1.

Let the student stand. Then slowly kneel down on the floor with one leg at a time. Then while kneeling down, let him slowly sit down on one side of his buttocks without help of his hands. He must never touch the ground with his hands.

2.

With infinite slowness the student will now lie down on the floor, placing the back, that is, each segment of the spine an inch at a time on the floor as he is lying down straight on the ground.

3.

Now let him reverse the process. Let the student infinitely slowly lift his head, neck, and back up to the waist so that every vertebrum stretches the ligaments between the vertebrae, by pulling the muscles of the back.

While doing this he must keep his mouth open and breathe through his mouth.

Here the physician must tell him not to take any more breath than is necessary for his normal breathing. In other words, he is not allowed to use oxygen "gas" through anxiety. The scientific meaning of it all is during this process of entire body oxidation, he should not be allowed to take any deep breathing. Therefore this mouth breathing.

The student must also be asked not to strain his eyes while working.

4.

In getting up on his knees, he shall very slowly stand up, kneeling first on one leg and getting up with the other leg until he is erect again.

5.

After the student slowly gets up, he slowly sits down again, folding one leg back (the left one if he has used the right one before) and slowly kneels down again until he is sitting down on the other side of his buttocks.

All this time he is not allowed to use his hands or arms at all, his arms and hands are being completely relaxed.

He should take this exercise ten or twelve times the first day and increase every day until he does it at least one hundred times a day to keep perfectly fit by beautiful, well-distributed circulation of blood and lymph fluid. The other physical training would be so much easier; the student will sleep soundly when he sleeps, and will digest and eliminate so normally that his life would be easy and happy.

The physician would observe that any psychological suggestion would hurt the student. It is the nerves and the protoplasm which will teach him happiness and not the application of new ideas to his brain. We must emphatically suggest to keep away from psychology and let all his ideas come from the secretions of the body—from the body to the brain and not from the brain to the body.

Shock-Proof Nerves

The average person knows that if he is going to bathe in a river or lake, he experiences a slight shock by the coolness of the water. This shock amounts to these physiological reactions: the person feels a little choking—he takes a gasp of breath and contracts the voluntary muscles of his body. In other words, he is fighting the coolness of the water, the sudden change in temperature, with his sympathetic nerves where his lungs and heart and the brain nerves are putting up the resistance and fight.

But if he had learned how to give up the resistance of the sympathetic nervous system and joyfully flow along the para-sympathetic lines, he would not receive the shock as much.

Similarly, when a student is trained physically to experience a fall by certain turning and twisting of the body violently and quickly, he is experiencing similar sympathetic nerve shocks. But when the student is trained along para-sympathetic lines, described in these exercises, it will be easier for him not to receive the shocks as much, and he will have iron-trained nerves.

Here is an example which will clarify our point.

Exercise v

Part One

1.

Every person knows the sensation of floating on the water. It is a feeling that permeates the whole body from the toe to the head.

Let the student learn to breathe through his mouth and bring about the feeling of floating in his body while he is sitting down, and later on when he is standing.

2.

He will never take any spasm of quick breath.

3.

He will never take deep breaths during all this training.

4.

Whensoever the student is considering any violent action with his nerves, he must guard against taking these gasps of breath, but bring about this floating feeling in his body on the very instant he institutes the physical action.

This is a new habit.

Part Two

The physician must give the student an example of quick violent form such as—

1.

Let the student fall on the ground as in a faint, with arms, legs, jaw and neck completely relaxed.

2.

During this moment the student will bring about the feeling of floating lightly and joyfully in his body—without fighting the breath.

In other words, the student's attention should be called to the oxygen supply. He must not use the oxygen "gas" very much. At no time of any sudden or violent action will he be allowed to use very much of this "gas" that is in the air.

It would be clear to him that this choking and violent action upsets the carbon dioxide balance and causes shock and exhaustion. Here mouth breathing would be good only because one cannot breathe so violently if the mouth is half open.

The Path

It is difficult to point out the practical implications of all these findings unless we establish a gigantic neurological laboratory where we show how man can resume the evolutionary path where he left off in the process of civilization or city building.

The corollaries of these findings are not academic. They will revolutionize our whole civilization. The schools and colleges and physical culture gymnasiums will become so revolutionized as to tend to give health and happiness and courage of life to mankind if we revive the heredity of the protoplasm rather than impose upon it by drug or cerebral ideas.

Our task is infinitely difficult because of the existing prejudices. Prize fighters of muscles and sympathetic nerves are training the muscle and sympathetic nerves of man. Cerebral workers known as psychologists are training the cerebrum of man. They are so far away from the river of life that life stands aside and laughs at man's poor attempt to improve himself.

We are introducing vitamin therapy after vitamin therapy to modify the protoplasm when the same protoplasm has gone through billions and trillions of countless years of evolution by seeking its own food and ingesting food wherever it has found it. The physiologist and neurologist have forgotten the capacity and the voltage of the organism—of the protoplasmic mass. They have forgotten the resistance of the protoplasmic mass also.

The news that we are giving herewith will be taken up a century hence by some future civilization if the modern educated man spits upon it today. With sincere affection in our heart and love of man we beg the biologists to study these facts of life in a very practical way by practical research.

Will not this revolutionize the science of medicine? Will this not upset our concept of internal medicine? Our whole new fount of cerebral architecture known as psychiatry? Will not this upset our whole system of child education? Take down the man on the high throne of college degrees and university prestige and status quo?

Here the protoplasm prays to its God silently to give it a chance for explosion and emanation of life. We pray with it that man will at least listen.

THIS PRECIOUS HEART

INTRODUCTION TO PART TWO

The heart when normal is a beautiful and very efficient pump, powerful and rhythmic in action. When pressure is needed it will increase in speed and force. The emergency ended, it slows down and rests. Naturally, like all muscles, when given unusual work it increases in size and power—the "athlete's heart."

The action of this pump, both as to power and rhythm, is controlled by two sets of nerves which we may liken, one to a conservative old man and the other to an excitable youth. One slows the heart and increases its power. The other insists on speeding it up. They usually balance one another and work more or less in harmony.

The heart is subject to certain diseases which tend to decrease its efficiency. Inflammatory conditions of its lining, from whatever cause, warp the valves and produce a leaky pump. This is a crippled but not a diseased heart. Often, especially in youth, this condition may slowly improve and result in a more or less perfect alignment of the valves and an efficient pump. Toxic substances in the blood produce over a long period of time a slow degeneration of all the cells in the heart, resulting in a true heart disease—a myocarditis—a permanently damaged organ and incurable.

But there are functional disturbances to the even rhythm of the heart which cause great distress to the body. These are disturbances of the nerves that control the rhythmic action of the pump. These may be due to mental and emotional explosions. They may be due to irritant chemical changes in the blood that supplies the energy to the heart muscle. Therefore, a philosophy of life which includes a mental and emotional discipline, which will give a patient the ability to relax and rest, will prevent in most cases these functional disturbances which are so wearing on this beautiful pump.

Pundit Acharya, who shows deep insight into the workings of

the human body and mind, does the layman a great service by explaining to him that a smooth level of consciousness is very vital to normalcy of life. These few lines from his book typify his whole attitude: "Human work and human thoughts always get the steam up in the physical and mental system. . . . You have a safety valve and that is your smile. As you smile, the constriction, blood pressure and heat of the body and the brain, all of the entire system cools down. Therefore, smile."

It is true, as the Pundit clearly points out, that a patient suffering from heart trouble should place himself at once in the hands of a competent physician, but here the Pundit starts with the individual before he becomes a patient. His is a biological approach that embraces the very rudiments of life chemistry. It is also true that the heart, like everything else, will eventually wear out, but under ideal conditions this most efficient pump should perform its function for one hundred and fifty years.

Thompson Sweeny, M.D.

A WORD

Softly I shall speak to the air.

The ears of man have become deaf with the sound of explosions. The eyes of man have become blind with tears.

By the scarred slopes and hills while innocent hearts fall asleep forever—

Gently, I shall speak to the air.

While quakes and eruptions terror the hearts of man, I shall retire to the depthless silence beyond the mind of man and repeat:

"Wherefore, whosoever shall eat this bread, and drink this cup of the Lord, unworthily, shall be guilty of the body and blood of the Lord."

The air into which I pour my heart shall permeate the hearts of Man.

I.

THE HEART

The heart is one of the most vital organs of the human body. Life itself depends upon the smooth and regular beats of the heart. When the heart fails, life fails with it.

In any medical library, one may read the pages on heart trouble in a book called: *Practice of Medicine* by Osler. Here one may find the varieties of heart trouble. The causes are many, and the treatments concern, mostly, slowing down the action of the heart, or stimulating the heart. But the sum total of all treatments will demand rest of the body and mind of the patient.

As one reads the pages, one will find that most of the patients suffering from chronic heart trouble should get ready to die sooner or later. In other words, anyone having heart trouble should expect death from heart failure any day. Of course the sufferer may live a long time with proper medical care and vigilance. But his heart will seldom be normal again. Nothing can really regenerate his heart and make it perfect.

Does it not give him a rather gloomy picture of life?

The picture is gloomier when we realize that the average life of complexity in civilization is such that it always invites heart trouble.

Jerky actions, twinging anxiety, chronic constipation, infectious diseases, irregular life, drunkenness, perfumed sensuality, etc., which are the abundant blessings of civilization, are some of the causes of heart trouble.

We are not writing a medical book and, therefore, we shall not deal with this phase of the story.

Because medicine is mostly concerned with heart trouble when it is already late for the heart to go back to normalcy, the physician treats a "cankered" heart. He does not and cannot afford to concern himself with the social process which sires the beginning of the heart trouble.

We shall go deep down, to life itself, to see where the heart finds its first trouble.

It is needless to say, anyone afflicted with the least suspicion of heart trouble should consult a doctor immediately, as neglect in this matter would be a question of life and death.

Brain of the Abdomen

Locate the end of the breast bone. Lying below it there is a mass of nerve fibers (celiac ganglion), which is called the abdominal brain. In other words, like the brain in the head, this brain of the abdomen controls the action of the heart, digestion, blood pressure, the lungs, the actions of the glands, and many of the nerves, and lastly, most of the emotions of the brain itself.

High blood pressure, hardening of the arteries, angina pectoris and other kinds of heart trouble are many times due to over-activity of this lower brain.

Heart trouble, starting with high blood pressure, is sometimes hereditary. That is, the cells inherit an over-activity of the lower brain of the abdomen.

In such cases, children have tremendous physical and mental activity during childhood, causing increasing tension, hardening of the arteries, etc., in middle or later life.

When the average person feels intensely emotional, and the heart is greatly disturbed, he sometimes has a sensation as though the blood flowing through the whole body and the brain, like a pool of water, has become muddy.

Have you not heard people say: "I feel sick to my stomach," after an emotional fit?

Often violent emotions such as hate, anger, fear, bring about this condition in the abdominal region, which the average person calls, "feeling sick to my stomach."

One of the greatest biologists and a noted surgeon, Dr. George Crile, finds operation on many of these nerve fibers of the abdominal brain causes a great relief to the person. Here are some of his public remarks:

"I would much rather have cancer than heart disease."

In his opinion, his operations in this part of the body have brought about "almost miraculous results" in the relief of heart pains, stopping of chronic headaches, and elimination of the general weakness and exhaustion, so charactertistic of various forms of the disease.

In a study of one hundred cases of angina pectoris, in which sharp, stabbing pains run all the way from the heart to the tips of the left fingers, the pain was stopped immediately by the operation. It has also proven highly successful in treating the dual problem of high blood pressure and partial stoppage of the coronary, the blood vessels which feed the heart itself.

Yoga Approach

We shall deal with the heart, and all the arteries leading into the heart, with a common sense approach.

We shall show the average person how to have a coordinated, regular, normal life of joy and happiness rather than pain and anxiety, so that he does not have heart trouble.

Please study this book carefully, and practice the exercises suggested in these pages.

Psychological advices from others or one's own thoughts will not teach anybody to control his heart.

The Yoga method is a physical method of utter simplicity, based upon reionization of the chemistry of the human body.

Mind is also body. Mind is made up of the brain cells. And when these brain cells work, the result is thoughts. Thoughts are merely the end products, that is, the leftover of brain actions. Thoughts cannot control thoughts. Thoughts cannot control the heart. Thoughts cannot cure heart trouble. Please remember this.

You will be the sorriest person on earth if you believe that we are giving psychological advice in this book. We are suggesting normalcy, depending upon normal functions of the body and the brain.

Heart Control means Sanity of Life.

Common Practices of Man

Here we start to look at man's activities and thoughts. We start to take pictures of his life. We avoid all technical complexities and speak simply, so that everybody can understand our language.

Let us be frank with ourselves. Let us take our own pictures. As we do, we find:

1. People who carry a cash register in their head have heart trouble. They should. Because they are the unthinking multitudes making up just the number of the species.

2. People who have to repress *pugnacity* every time they talk to someone have heart trouble. (Watch two people talking. Each one is waiting impatiently—although through courtesy withholding the tongue—to say his say. Each one is a teacher in a world of teachers where there are not very many students. During this waiting time one is in agony because he cannot talk and drown the other out. Do you think he is listening to the words of the other fellow in great ecstasy of relaxation and gratitude? No. He is fuming inside with carbon dioxide.)

3. People who criticize and analyze everything in life do never enjoy the flow and romance of life. They are the Chanticleers without whose crowing the sun cannot rise. They would take the blocks of a building apart to see if there be any roaches inside. They do have and should have heart trouble.

4. People who always blame their accursed fate or others for their own failures and disappointments have heart trouble.

5. People who feel the pangs of hate, generating fumes of venom within, have heart trouble.

6. People who feel anger in all its shades and tones, or are constantly vexed, have heart trouble.

7. People who suffer from unavenged revenge, for wrongs done to either themselves or to their nation or race, have heart trouble.

8. People who pity themselves continually, jealous of others' opportunities and successes, have heart trouble.

9. People who suffer from the scorpion stings of jealousy, envy and greed have heart trouble.

10. People who suffer from waspishness, sticking out branches of their vanity all around their personality, so that anybody can hurt their susceptible, sensitive nature, have heart trouble.

11. People who believe in real or imaginary enemies have heart trouble.

12. People who are afraid, ranging from fear of the boss to the fear of death, have heart trouble.

13. People who worry, and always seek and find causes of worry, have heart trouble.

14. People who "rush in" with anxiety and "gush in" with enthusiasm to think or do things, have heart trouble.

15. People whose mouths are tight with stingy thoughts and over-cautiousness have heart trouble.

16. People whose body is stiff and unbending and petrified have heart trouble.

17. People who have lost the sense of childish play have heart trouble.

18. People who are born constitutionally unhappy have heart trouble.

19. People who have nothing, outside of themselves, to live for, have heart trouble.

20. People who live for personal ambitions, not knowing whether they want to be Napoleon or Nelson, Galli Curci or Joan of Arc, have heart trouble.

21. People who cannot surrender—surrender to the simplicity of "Thy Will be done"—have heart trouble.

22. People who are smart, intellectually and socially brilliant, and are not mellow aesthetically and spiritually, have heart trouble.

23. People whose happiness does not flow out from the spring of bearing the cross for the greatest good of humanity, have heart trouble.

24. People who are nothing but thoughts and thoughts and more thoughts, and who live on their emotions, have heart trouble.

25. Men and women and even children who have never learned to bend their head to the dust in prayer do and should have heart trouble.

One should ask why—

The Why of It

Here is the picture of the inside of the body and mind which will answer most of these questions. Please read patiently:

The heart is like a pump which pushes the blood from itself to the lungs for two reasons:

1. To get rid of the poison of the body—carbon dioxide.

2. To take fresh oxygen from the lungs.

The heart pushes the fresh, oxidized blood to the rest of the body and the brain. Again the heart "sucks" the "filthy blood" from the body into its own valves and sends it to the lungs to be purified.

Without this purified blood life cannot go on for a minute.

Anything that stops this holy purification of the blood will cause the death of the heart and life.

Now, watch yourself.

The moment you are holding your breath with a jerk of a movement—that moment you are killing yourself. That is the beginning of Heart Trouble.

Can we make it any simpler?

In one word we ask you this question. Every time you start to think, talk, or act, do you not put a cork in your nose and mouth so no fresh air can get into your lungs?

We further ask you the question, do you think that in that moment the blood can be purified?

We further ask you the question, what do you think has happened to the lungs and the heart in that moment? What has happened to the miles of arteries and veins and all the tubings carrying the blood and the lymph?

Here is our whole story.

In our exercises given later in this book, we show how the average man can regulate his thoughts and actions every hour of the day in such a way as not to fight with his breath and heart.

One would ask the question, how on earth can a man move, act, walk, think, without disturbing his regular breathing process and the flow of blood that the heart has to pump?

Here we give you an immortal and a precious rule which will be the salvation of mankind if they understand it and faithfully live up to it.

We are asking you to revive the *Bird in Man*. A feathery existence through flowing days and nights.

This bird movement of the human body and mind should be like the scaling of the air by the wings of a bird. This scaling of the air must be felt by the nerves of the body.

In other words, as a man shall move, walk, turn a corner, think, he shall feel as though his body and mind are floating in the air. Every time he shall make a turn he shall feel the sensation of yawning during turning and moving—as in languor.

It is this feeling alone in the movement of the body and the thoughts of the mind which will keep his lungs and heart cool and regular.

Man has forgotten his heredity of the reptile and the bird kingdom. The agility of the serpentine and feline kingdom. So his body has become stiff. Man has forgotten the dance of life. So his body has become ugly.

Biologists cannot tell us that the cells and the nerves and the glands of the body of man and even the brain of man have forgotten to inherit these past experiences of life.

We will not quarrel with the biologists, nor will we start any discussion with them. We shall take it for granted that biology of tomorrow will come up to the level of our intuition. We shall not try to educate biology to understand this.

It is up to the man to revive the bird in him and the feline in him.

The only way he will do it is through his feeling during his movements, and not while he is sitting down and figuring it out. That is, when he is making a turn, lifting a leg, getting up or sitting down; and in all his movements, he shall feel the feeling of scaling the air by the wings of a bird.

This will keep his heart calm. Because he will not bring jerky, muscular contraction in his body during action.

This thing should be taught early in life, from the very time the children learn to walk. In fact in all the grammar schools of the world before the body of the little ones become stiff enough to kill the heart.

Herewith we examine the average man and see what he is doing, and then we shall give him the exercises with explanations.

Action Samples

Watch an expressman lift a very heavy package. He does not pick it up straight. He gives it a swing, and with an exhalation of his breath, at the very moment of the swing, he lifts the package to his shoulder.

One would ask, why does he not pick it up straight? Why does he swing it in lifting it up to his shoulder?

The answer is the very revelation of life to humanity. If humanity would stop right here and think. He is unconsciously escaping the gravity of the earth by exhaling his breath as he lifts the heavy package. If he only knew it!

Watch, on the other hand, the average person lift something heavy.

He holds his breath, contracts the most of the muscles of the body, including the back of his neck and the nerves of his eyes. The average person holds his breath, and fights gravity with all his might. He bears the brunt of the whole weight of the package that he is lifting, as he lifts it straight.

One may easily see how the average person is actually fighting with the thing he has to lift. Here he is actually fighting gravity, the pain of human existence.

Now suppose this average person learned to swing the thing a little, like the expressman, and pick it up with an exhalation of his breath, rather than holding the breath. And suppose he brought a sense of play along with the work and smiled.

If he did, he would find the weight of the package become light with the exhalation of his breath. He would further find that all the muscles of his body would not be contracted as much. Nor would he have to fight his breath.

Ordinarily, persons picking up packages and doing heavy work all day long are fighting gravity and friction.

This is the beginning of his heart trouble which he does not know. Nor do the leaders of thought of mankind ever tell him this.

Later on, it will be shown, from the simple laws of physics, that the most of the time human energy is being spent in fighting gravity and friction causing strain on the heart, fatigue, exhaustion, and finally death.

In this book, exercises will be given to the average person which will teach him how to escape this gravity and friction, so that he can go on working all day long without very much strain on his heart.

In the meantime we shall examine how this fighting with gravity in heavy work really causes the beginning of the heart trouble.

Here we quote Dr. Willian Osler, one of the greatest men in the field of internal medicine. Speaking of Chronic Valvular Disease

—Aortic Incompetency—he says in his book, *Practice of Medicine*:

"By far the most frequent cause of insufficiency is the slow, progressive sclerosis of the segment, resulting in a curling of the edge, which lessens the working surface of the valve. This may, of course, follow acute endocarditis, but it is so often met with in strong, able-bodied men among the working classes without any history of rheumatism or special febrile disease with which endocarditis is commonly associated, that other conditions must be sought for to explain its frequency. Of these, unquestionably, strain is the most important—not of a sudden, forcible strain, but a persistent increase of the normal tension to which the segments are subject during the diastole of the ventricle. Of circumstances increasing this tension, heavy and excessive use of the muscles is perhaps the most important. So often is this form of heart disease found in persons devoted to athletics that it is sometimes called the 'athlete's heart.' Alcohol is a second important factor, and is stated to raise considerably the tension of the aortic system. A combination of these two causes is extremely common."

Simple Laws of Physics

Now we are giving a simple law of Physics. We quote from *Practical Physics* by Robert Andrews Millikan, Ph. D. and Sc. D., and Henry Gordon Dale, Ph. D.

"The work done by acting forces is equal to the sum of the kinetic and potential energies stored up."

In other words, if there be any friction on the path of the work, much of the work is wasted. The law is: *Friction always Results in Wasted Work.*

To make it very plain, if a machine is going on without any friction, it will do a certain amount of work. But if something stands in its way, causing friction, resulting from some resistance, a lot of energy of the machine will be wasted, and its efficiency will be decreased.

The same law holds good with regard to human energy and work.

If a person is working with his energy in a very smooth way, that is, if there is no friciton, his energy will carry on the work efficiently without wasting any part of it. But if he has friction, he will have to spend more energy to do the same amount of work, which he could have done smoothly with less energy, had he had no friction.

Later on, it will be shown that it is *this friction* which is the waste of action and thoughts of man and which finally causes him all the trouble. This is the beginning of his heart trouble.

In another chapter it will also be shown how this friction is the cause of bad digestion, poor elimination and loss of vitality. Still farther, it will be shown how human happiness itself is dependent upon actions of the body and the mind without friction.

The object of this work is to take out the jerks and creases and sands from the path of thoughts and actions of the average man, so that his life process may flow on smoothly like the flow of a river.

In our book, *A Strange Language*, we have predicted:

"Life shall be a smile forever."

Thought Samples

Now we shall examine the thinking and acting processes of the average man. To see how he not only wastes his energy and loses his efficiency of life itself, but how he brings about a condition which begins to tell on his heart.

Watch somebody sit down and do a little serious thinking. The most of the time he is day dreaming. Or perhaps he is retrospecting. Or perhaps he is getting an ambitious idea. Or still further, perhaps he is thinking about all the things that he has done in the past, and so on.

You will notice with every thought in his brain he is getting a sudden motor impulse. This motor impulse, being translated into some muscles of his body, is causing muscular contraction. He is moving his eyeballs without being conscious of it. He is straining his eye nerves as he is mentally localizing things and happenings in mental places. In other words, he is "doing things" without knowing.

As he thinks, he lives through situation after situation. This is bringing about tense motor impulses in his brain. They are going through all the muscles of his body. In other words, the sensory and motor nerves of his body are sending spasmodic currents of electricity from his brain to the body and again from the body (muscles, etc.) to the brain. All these jerky currents are sending jerky nerve impulses to the heart.

Thus, to all intent and purpose, his thinking is causing spasmodic muscular contractions and relaxations alternately. This he does not know.

It will be shown in this study of the beatings of the heart, how all muscular contractions are the cause of heart excitement.

It will be further shown in the study how these unrhythmic, spasmodic, jerky contractions of the muscles, due to these chaotic actions of the human brain, are the beginning of heart trouble.

But let us go on further with our story.

You will notice that the thinking person, that is, the person playing havoc with his thoughts, is sometimes taking a gaspy, deep breath and holding it too long. Then at other times he is giving out a quick sharp breath. His breath is working in jerky, gaspy spasms. His thoughts mean jerky breaths.

Not for one moment will you find the thinking man taking a relaxed and regular, easy breath.

Heart and lungs are sister organs. One may easily see that when the one works, the other also works; and when the one rests, the other rests also. The trouble with the lungs spells the trouble with the heart. Rest of the lungs means rest of the heart.

We saw how the man "in thought" is having trouble with his lungs: meaning he is breathing in gasps. Therefore, it is easy to see that he is having irregular beats of the heart along with his irregular breathing. This will be shown more clearly a little later on.

We shall go a little deeper into our story. Watch someone who is going out to a play or to some pleasure. If one observes very minutely, one finds that when he is going out to enjoy himself; while he is walking and thinking, "window-wishing" and watching things, he is continually taking irregular breaths. That is to say, all the while he is going to enjoy himself, he is hurting himself with irregular breathing.

You would also notice that he is having "pit-a-pat" contraction and relaxation of his muscles alternately in the process of his thinking and hoping to enjoy.

One may ask, if one is going to enjoy, that is, be happy, why one should cause panting of his lungs and throbbing of his heart?

The answer is that in his childhood days he has formed these habits. Because nobody taught him any better.

Life is a dance. A rhythmic flow. As everything in the universe is in perfect rhythm. Man alone violates this universal law of rhythm in his walking, talking, moving, thinking, playing, dreaming – day or night–night or day.

Strength, No Guarantee against Heart Trouble

Now we shall take the case of a perfectly healthy man. A strong man. A giant of a man or woman. We shall talk about a prize fighter or wrestler.

Every time the prize fighter is making up his mind to gather up all his physical energy in the muscles of his arms, he is fixing his attention on some spot of the body of the enemy that he is going to hit.

Stop right there and examine what he is doing.

He is going through a mental process which is causing his jaws to set, all the muscles of his body to contract. His eye nerves and the eyeballs are feeling the pressure of contraction. His head (blood pressure) is getting hot.

What do you think is happening to his lungs and heart at this time? That is, with the very birth of the idea that he has to gather up the energy to fight?

Now he launches a blow. Next, he gets ready for the next blow, and so on. So during the entire process of his fight, the strong man, the ideal man of strength, is playing havoc with his heart.

The Science of Medicine tells us he will die of heart trouble, that is, of "athlete's heart."

Again, what about the thousands who are watching the prize fight? Gasping and screaming and yelling and convulsing in the worst kind of War Hysteria!

Now let us go to a ball game.

We are in the grandstand. The players in the field are getting into different positions. Now they are playing with the ball: picking it up, snatching it from the opposite side, and making a dash. While they are practically going on with different phases of the play—watch the people in the grandstand.

These people are playing the game by proxy along with the players, who are actually engaged in the game. Through the process of "idio-motor" reactions, the proxy players are going through the play just the same as the players, so far as the nerves and muscles are concerned. The players at least have the release of the play. But the proxy players are only enjoying the spasms of hysteria. What a hell to the poor heart!

In other words, the nerves and muscles of the body of these sightseers are getting excited. But having no ball or opposite party to get response from, they remain unsated. Thus they are going through a nervous and physical tension of the worst kind.

As we shall study what excites and what calms the heart, we shall see how they are playing football with their hearts. Not only the players but also those in the grandstand who have bought tickets to the funeral of their heart.

Every time they get excited, they are holding their breaths and choking. The next moment they are exhaling the breath violently. And the next moment they are taking another deep, violent breath. And along with this violent breathing in and out, their heart is jumping and thumping violently, crying for a release. When the game is over they are all tired out, and you may easily see the condition of their hearts.

In youth when the vitality is very great, they do not know what has happened to their hearts. They use this motor in such a way in their youth that, as they get older, they find their motor failing.

Then they blame the doctor for not being able to repair the motor.

Now let us go and take a ride in a subway or a bus.

With every turn and twist of the train of the car, it is making a squeaking and screeching sound. With every turn and twist it is crashing and banging as though, from the heart of the inferno, the very jaws of hell are yelling out with crashing noise. Every sudden jamming of the brakes to stop and every lurching turn of the bus is causing a violent jerk of the body.

The nerves of the body are sending impulses to the muscles, making them dance and re-dance, jump and twist and turn as the car is doing on the road. One may easily see what is happening to the heart!

In other words, jerk after jerk is going on inside of the body and the brain of the person "enjoying" the subway or bus ride. It has been noticed that often children when first riding in a street car or bus become sick to their stomach.

These muscular sensations to and from the brain are playing upon the heart.

If one could translate the sounds of the heart, as one does in a   —
psychological laboratory, one would hear such chaotic beating of drums that one would be horrified to know the effect of the bus or subway sounds upon himself.

Not only that. The eyeballs and the nerves of the eyes and the retina are correspondingly played upon, with the result that one is losing eyesight along with it.

Let us now find a luxurious city apartment where a person has at last gone to sleep, to rest. Somewhere, near one of the fashionable streets of the metropolis.

As one is about to fall asleep, all of a sudden, a heavy motor truck crashes through the streets, or some joy riders coming from a night club make a savage noise. The sleeper's heart goes a-fluttering. One is dazed: doesn't know what has happened.

Now, all of a sudden the police siren or the fire siren gives a hellish, screeching noise in the street and the half-sleepy heart, terror-stricken, jumps up with a scream. The person who was but half asleep and going to the other land of rest!

This noise came so suddenly and abruptly, like the explosion of a bomb, that the person could not come back to consciousness so quickly. The result was, the heart and lungs and the rest of the body had to make an adjustment too quickly.

One may easily see how civilization thus stabbed the sleepy heart. A wound, that later on, the civilization will try to cure with drops of digitalis.

We have given some of the inside pictures showing how jerky, sudden actions and thoughts, causing frictions, disturb the very flow of life. It is the disturbance of Life Flow, the flow of blood and lymph, which causes the pumping of the heart, sometimes violently, and at other times subnormally, when one is exhausted.

Instead of dealing with the story any farther, we first give you the exercises, and a little later on shall give further explanations.

II.

HEART EXERCISES

Exercise i
Experiencing Sensory Sensation

1.

Sit down calmly. Feel relaxed as much as possible. Infinitely slowly, still more slowly, start to yawn, using all the muscles of the body from the waist up. Even if you have to make sounds as "ah," "oo" with your yawning.

2.

As you yawn, try to feel the sensation of the muscles. Do not imagine the sensation, but feel the thrill of the sensation of yawning in the muscles. This is sensory enjoyment. In yawning, do not try to stretch the muscles with volition and fight, but try to make them feel like a piece of cotton.

3.

You would say: "I cannot distinguish the sensory enjoyment from the motor impulse. Or I cannot stop watching the sensation with my mind." Very well.

4.

Imagine the sourness of a very sour lemon. Now, where do you feel the sourness? Is it not through your whole body that you feel the shiver of sourness? In the nerves and muscles of the body? As one can feel the sourness of a lemon, so one can feel the sweetness of a lump of sugar throughout the whole body. Here one learns how to feel sensations through the whole body.

5.

Now, as you yawn again, taste the sweetness of the sensation of a languorous, lazy, dishevelling, slow yawning. As you taste sweet things with your mouth, so you taste the sensation with your body. Feel the sugar of the burning glycogen stored up in the muscles of the body. Glycogen is carbohydrate or sugar. As you are using the muscles in yawning, you are actually burning up sugar.

Feel this sugar as you felt the lemon, with the same kind of a thrill. Do not imagine it. Do not put mind over matter. Give your mind a vacation. Don't think it, but taste it. Enjoy it through the waves of your body.

6.

Now start very slowly. Begin a thin smile on your lips.

7.

Now as you smile more, while yawning, send this smile through the nerves and sinews, and let this smile flow slowly through the blood of your body.

8.

Feel the smile in all parts of your body from head to foot.

9.

Do it at least fifty times a day. Only be very sure that you do not use much effort. Your attention should be toward Languor and Release and Enjoyment, rather than Effort and Fiat and Volition.

10.

As the muscles of your body are smiling, giving you the thrill of a feline movement, they will send sensory sensations to the back of the neck of your body, where the cardiac inhibitory center will be stimulated and the nerves will send a sweet, pleasant sensation of relaxation to the muscles of the heart. Thus the heart will learn to rest.

Warning: We know that you will *try* to do this thing. Please, we beg of you, do not try with your mind, but you yourself feel this sensation, and do not try to do anything with effort or volition, that is, by thinking processes. Here you have to come away from thinking to the feeling kingdom.

Exercise ii
Relaxation of the Neck

Part One

1.

Sit comfortably in a chair. Take a deep breath slowly. Exhale slowly. Do not try to think or fret and fidget now.

2.

Turn your neck slowly, moving a fraction of an inch at a time. Feel and enjoy the sensation of the muscles. The idea is to loosen the control of the neck the same as an infant has no control of the neck.

3.

Slowly loosen the energy that it takes to hold the neck up.

4.

Make the neck limp, like a piece of rag, as though the neck and the head do not belong to you.

5.

Drop the neck. Drop it in front, side, back, dropping and turning it at the same time, slowly, infinitely slowly, and keep on enjoying the sensation of losing it. As you do this, you will notice your heart is calming down and you will feel drowsy.

Part Two

6.

Now lie down calmly in bed and try to loosen the neck in the same way.

7.

Do not fight, but move along and downward, sloping toward drowsiness and peace as the sense of rest is coming.

8.

Do not arouse fight, effort and thinking. As soon as new thinking, that is, thoughts are coming into the brain, smile gently and give up and move along with the approach of sleep.

You will notice your heart is becoming calm.

Part Three

9.

The first few days or weeks you take this exercise, you will fall asleep.

10.

Gradually you shall have learned during the day how to loosen your neck, instead of having tightness there, and feeling heat in the head.

In this way you shall have learned how to keep your heart calm and you shall have learned not to worry or suffer from sleeplessness or restlessness at night.

Explanation

Years ago a man named Mr. Mesmer invented a method called Mesmerism to bring about hypnosis, that is, sleep in people.

That is, he gave a very gentle soft massage on the neck and the base of the head near the base of the brain to relieve the pressure.

Now by so doing he found out that the rate of flow of blood in the brain becomes low as he gives the sensory sensation to the muscles and indirectly to the nerves of the back of the neck.

Here, without a second party giving a massage on the neck, you are learning to bring about a very pleasant, delicate, sensuous sensation in the back of your neck by your work of loosening the neck as an infant wiggles his neck without any control. When you shall have made your neck like a piece of rag, you will have found this sweet, sensuous enjoyment.

This process has stimulated the cardiac inhibitory center in the neck the same as digitalis does by stimulating the pneumogastric nerves or vagii.

Here, through the Yoga method, the individual learns how to enjoy his sensory sensations and give a vacation to his motor reactions and motor impulses: thoughts that are aroused by the process of thinking and worrying and trying to do something.

The layman must learn this once for all, and keep on learning, until he has formed these habits, and such habits have become his second nature, so that he will never try to do things, but float along with the sensation, and enjoy life.

Enjoyment of such a sensation alone will calm down his heart and give it a rest.

The heart of the average person, God knows, knows no rest. This will save the lives of millions of mankind.

Exercise iii
Cooling the System

The third set of exercises consists of two common sense practices to form a new habit, so that one may keep as normal as humanly possible.

Every steam boiler has a water-cooling system. The automobile has a radiator to keep the motor cool. Nature has given water to two-thirds of the human body to keep the human body cool. There is even a water cooler in the brain to keep the brain cool. Every cell of the body as well as the brain has water in it to keep it cool.

Therefore nature demands that one learn to use this water-cooling system of the body and mind.

Part One

1.

During your daily work or during your thinking or emotional

states of mind, catch yourself at any given moment and feel the temperature sense of your body and the brain. And, by the following method, try to cool down your body and the brain by releasing the breath and smiling. One must always keep one's body and brain cool. This should be a new habit.

2.

Feel slowly–a smile, with a sense of play, humor and release– and bring about coolness inside the body and the brain.

Everybody has a thermal sense of the body. Meaning one can feel the heat or the coolness of the whole body. Now, smile and loosen up as in yawning and you will feel the body getting cooler. Remain cool.

The aim is not to keep cool, as they say, but *feel* cool.

3.

As soon as you are getting hot, either through work or through thoughts, your normalcy is being upset. Immediately see to it that you bring the coolness back. Human work and human thoughts always get the steam up in the physical and mental system. If you have too much steam you will burst the boiler. The boiler in this case is your central nervous system.

4.

You have a safety valve and that is your smile. As you smile, the constriction, blood pressure, and heat of the body and the brain, all of the entire system cools down. Therefore, smile.

Part Two

When you wake up in the morning you find a balanced state in your body and mind. In other words, you have not generated any heat through thoughts and actions as you do during the day.

Now as you proceed to work and think, you are getting up your energy or steam and spending it.

The food that you eat, especially carbohydrates or starchy food, gives you energy of the body and the brain. In action and in thought you are continually using up this energy. When all the energy is used up, you are fatigued and nervous, and the heart is "played out." In such a case food alone will not restore your energy, because your very tired body and mind are not conducive to digestion.

The fatigue stage shows that the balance between the body energy and the outside world has been upset. (This has upset the "carbon balance.")

Now you start to re-establish or bring back this balance. You will do it in this way.

1.

Sit down for about five minutes and exhale, or breath out slowly, by throwing out the carbon dioxide from inside your lungs. Make these exhalations, Short and Simple. Beware—

2.

As you do it, see that you do not make any effort or fight with the breath and cause friction. But slowly, and very gently, breathe out as much as you can.

3.

In breathing out, take the abdominal cavity in, and get rid of as much air as possible by slow breathing out. Only do not try to breathe out all the air from the lungs, but just enough consistent with ease of the body. This is very important.

4.

But the most important thing to remember here, when you are breathing out, is to give off the physical energy and tightness and thoughts from the brain *as* you breathe out.

5.

To do this, naturally you have to smile with a sense of humor and play. This will refresh you and you will re-establish or bring back the balance.

In other words, you will again feel refreshed, just as you did when you got up from your bed in the morning.

6.

Do this exhalation and feel light for five minutes several times during the day. It is like stopping the motor of an automobile after a two-hundred or three-hundred mile drive and letting the machine cool for half an hour.

You do not need a long rest, but you need two or three minutes' rest at a time between your work and between your complex and emotional "thinking."

These little breakwaters will keep up your energy indefinitely, and here you will learn how to rest your body and mind and therefore your heart.

Exercise iv
Depressed Heart

There is another condition which will cause heart trouble eventually in any human being, and that is depression.

You know that extreme fear which threatens the very life of the human being will paralyze the body, and almost stop the heart beat, for a few seconds.

You also know that extreme grief, when you feel as though you have lost everything in life, will also bring about a sense of paralysis of the body and the mind, slowing down the heart beat.

These are extreme cases.

Similarly, all despair, all disappointments, all blasted hopes will bring about a state of mind which will drag the mental energy to a point lower than the level of life.

Here the heart will suffer a depression, with such low and feeble beats, which will not be its rest at all, but will be a very unhealthy subnormal condition for the organ of the heart.

Just as abrupt and violent beats of the heart will wear out the heart in the long run, so also a very depressed condition of the heart will stop its normal work and rest.

Hope and happiness, a sense of play, and release, and peace of mind and body, are the necessary conditions for a normal heart.

If you are ever in such a state of depression:

1.

Sit down calmly in a place, and very slowly, infinitely slowly, start to stretch your body, and start yawning.

2.

We know in such a state of depression of the mind, you cannot possibly smile very easily. But, as you are stretching and yawning, try to feel the ease of the body coming back.

3.

Do not yawn or stretch abruptly. But by gradual, slow degrees, start to stretch the muscles and ligaments and sinews of the body, and take slowly, and slowly, deeper, and deeper breaths. Meaning inhalation and exhalation.

4.

Do not think, but keep on breathing in and out with every turn and twist, and stretch and yawn with the whole body. But do not tire yourself. This will restore the normalcy slowly but surely.

5.

Do not create any false hopes artificially by thinking, because if the cause of the depression is still there, no thoughts will ever inspire you enough to take you out of the depression.

Grief and fear and despair have caused an acid condition in your body. That is, the whole body is filled with poisonous end products.

You must neutralize this poisonous condition by giving oxygen to every part of the body, and relieve the tension of the muscles caused by the slumping of the body through grief and despair and this negative state of mind.

Oxygen, here, is the medicine which will neutralize the poison.

You must read the section entitled "Breath Is Life," which will teach you how to breathe through your palms and feet and the whole body joyously.

Exercise v
Feeling of Lightness

The average person fights the pull of the earth, the weight of things, and through his thoughts he fights mentally also.

This is the birth of friction. All energy used in working is wasted through friction. These are very simple laws of practical physics that we learn in our high school days.

Therefore one should learn here how to act and think all day long without this friction.

In this slow breathing out, feel you are giving up the load of life. To the average person the sense of the muscles of the body is like a heavy bundle. As you breathe out, you will give it up to the earth.

Close your eyes, take note of the weight of your body. You feel so many pounds. As you breathe out give up these pounds, and as you come out with a smile in breathing out, feel like a feather. Be light in the head and the upper part of your body.

Feel this giving up. Don't think it.

This exercise will teach you how to develop a new habit, so that on a moment's notice you will learn to give up, "dust to dust," and come out with a smile. Be a bird-man.

This would be for the first time a knowledge, and not a thought, that you are that smile, and not the heaviness which you feel as you fight matter and mind.

1.

Sit quietly somewhere.

2.

Slowly, infinitely slowly, by graduated degrees, breathe out all the air you possibly can. Only do not constrict your neck, face, eyes by violent effort. Beware. Breathe out as though you are taking the air out from the legs, thighs, abdomen, lungs, muscles and the whole body. As though you are taking all the refuse matter from the entire body and throwing it out in the process of exhalation. As though you are taking out all the carbon dioxide as you breathe out. Slowly. Beware.

3.

You would ask, how can you possibly pull out all the carbon dioxide?

Bring a sense of pulling, and feel the stirring up of all the muscles of the body in breathing out. As though you are bringing up the foul air from all parts of the body. Through exhalation, in this process of pulling, you are vitalizing the whole body.

4.

Now, as you exhale by *graduated degrees*, and slowly give up the fight of life, meaning tightness, tension, stiffness, and the sense of fiat or volition (what you call will), you are feeling a sense of dropping off of the whole weight of your life. That is, when you "flop," "slump," with every exhalation.

That which belongs to gravity, you are giving up to gravity; and you are coming out of it nudely with a bare smile.

That smile is you. That is what you call your soul.

A few times of this breathing out from head to foot, so long as you do not stir up your body with fight and tension again, will have taught you how to enjoy these senses of your body.

Here is the honey of life, the elixir of happiness, and the release of the heart.

This practice, all the while, will give you relaxation of the heart.

Exercise vi
Complete Relaxation

Part One

1.

Sit quietly in a chair. Place your left hand on your lap. See that you feel no resistance.

2.

Feel as though your hand does not belong to you. Make it lifeless. Give up owning the hand. Let it feel heavy. As though the hand belongs to somebody else.

3.

Try to lift the left hand by the right hand. Hold the left by the thumb and let it fall on your lap. Let it fall down on the lap limp.

4.

Keep on feeling limp until you feel the left hand absolutely lifeless.

Part Two

5.

Now, after you have found the left hand completely gone, as though there is no more life left in it, (although the rest of the body is under your control), try to feel the whole left arm, starting from the shoulder, also gone. That is, lose control of it the same way as you do of the hand.

6.

As the whole left arm, hand and all, has become numb and heavy, shake your head a little and see that you yourself, meaning your own consciousness, are not drowsy.

7.

This is called hypnosis of the arm and hands, or local hypnosis.

8.

You must try this in one part of the body at a time, after you have succeeded in completely losing the sense of owning the arm and the hand. That is, when the whole arm has become completely limp, heavy and lifeless.

9.

Lie down and bring this sense of loss all over the body except *the head*, meaning your consciousness.

10.

So that you do not hypnotize yourself and feel drowsy, please keep a vague smile in your consciousness and keep the brain clear. Only, do not stir anything in the body.

11.

You will find that your body is perfectly still. That is, your heart, lungs, and all other organs of the body are hibernating. The whole body is working very nicely and normally internally without interference of your mind.

Part Three

12.

So far as the mind is concerned, do not bring thoughts and stir up the body. In other words, do not start any motor impulses. Here you shall learn to rest in a sweet smile, and you shall practice this whenever necessary to gain control over your whole body.

Part Four

13.

Do not practice this in such a way that you will feel your brain also numb and lazy. As soon as you feel sleepy, smile. Keep on smiling, more smile, more, and you shall have a very clear brain while the body is asleep.

14.

Do not fear that if you fall asleep in practicing these exercises you will harm yourself. It will be a very sweet sleep and no harm will come to you.

15.

In learning to bring about local hypnosis in any part of the body, you—meaning your mind—should remain on the side of gentleness.

16.

All the practices in this book demand that you do these things with infinite slowness. Because the objective of all these exercises is to teach you how to enjoy the flow of life, meaning the flow of the blood and the lymph fluid.

Part Five

17.

One cannot go immediately from a rose garden to a sewer, and still keep the beauty and fragrance of the rose garden in his senses. Similarly, after you shall have experienced this peaceful and blissful state, do not jump up with a jerk or hurry and start to beat the hellish drums of modern civilization. Remain floating on the smile and honey of life and learn to pay no attention to the Coyotes of Society.

18.

Carry the soft and gentle, peaceful and blissful state of mind, where there is no strain or tightness or tension, into the rest of the day. That is, as you work, move, think, keep this gentleness all over your body all day long. At night you will have a dreamless sweet sleep. You will wake up in a beautiful morning the next day.

This will teach you how to form a new habit where the heart will control itself.

Life is a soft crooning flow of a river of milk and honey, where smiles shall foam out to the rays of the sun, which are the solar energy of life given by the god of the sun.

Life, the eternal river, distributes happiness and delight on both shores, giving life, the life energy to everything that falls on its path.

Life, the river, has come from the waterfall of unseen life and is bound for the infinite unbound sea, the depthless deep of life.

Life, the river, is a river of beauty, ravished and dishevelled from within, and laughing forever outwardly the joys of being and going to the infinite and nameless sea, its destiny.

Exercise vii
Essence of Smiles

This exercise, the surest cure of all heart trouble, is the smile of happiness.

This smile is not the smile of a salesman, or of a social butterfly, to coquette the other fellow's heart, so that the other fellow will be beguiled and give a sweet response.

This smile must come out and rise out from every nerve cell and muscle cell of the body and the mind. This smile must be an explosion of the "Amiya," (The Nectar), in the cells of the body.

You must learn therefore to teach the cells of the body, which are like animals of a zoo, to smile and enjoy.

This smile of enjoyment is the birth of happiness.

This is the training for a new life.

One who has been fortunate enough to train one's body and mind to smile with his entire body, has tasted the real secret nectar of life. We have called this "Amiya."

No one could ever bring about this smile and happiness in the muscles and nerves of the body by imagining it.

This takes one to one's feeling world.

Here one must learn, once for all, without any question or suspicion or inquiry or analysis, how to feel the thrill that one does out of these smiles of the cells of the body. Cell smile and cell happiness will save your heart trouble.

Hate, anger, disgust, apathy, vengeance, fear and worry, continual criticism and analysis of things in life, and similar mental processes kill the heart. They kill the heart by generating cell secretions in the brain and the body which are poisonous in nature.

One might easily assume that extreme hate or pugnacity for years and years would make the cells of the body secrete a peculiar type of aminoacid which perhaps is the beginning of cancer.

Hate and the spirit of vengeance and venomous emotions which go with cancer, are certainly enough to kill the heart. You cannot trample upon the hearts of others and go without having heart trouble yourself. You cannot smother others' hearts and feel peace and happiness in your own heart.

Shrewd and cunning men and women make a million and go to bed with a grin of satisfaction that they have successfully robbed many ignorant and poor workingmen. They wake up the next morning with indigestion and heart burn. They call their doctor.

But what doctor can prescribe more than: "The price of sin is death."

The Need of Training

The entire process of heart control depends primarily upon control of the afferent, incoming sensations to and from the brain.

To make it more explicit, one has to learn how to control the sensations coming from the muscles of the body, and passing through the back of the neck (the medulla oblongata), and going to the brain; and also the sensations coming from the brain, and going through the back of the neck (the medulla oblongata), to the rest of the body.

Every sensation has four properties: namely, extensity, intensity, quality, and tone.

In the control of these afferent sensations one cannot very well stop the sensations from coming to and from the brain. What one actually can do therefore is *not to receive* the tremendous intensity of the sensations, as these sensations arrive.

This one can do by receiving as little intensity as is humanly possible.

The method is Release.

Did you not see the expressman lift the weight as he exhaled? He released the muscles and general tension through exhaling. By exhaling of the breath also, he refused to accept as much intensity of the muscular tension as he would have received had he not exhaled and given the swing to the package.

Similarly, one may easily see that as one is going to rest, and is falling asleep, one does not accept as much noise, light and other sensations of the muscles; that is, from the eye nerves, ear nerves, and so on; and one does not give as much motor response to the stimuli.

Do you see how one may keep his mind in a state of smiling and laughing—in a state of happiness that is, in a word, Release, so that one does not accept full intensity of any sensation coming to the brain?

One could learn to be too busy with bliss and peace to receive a sensation in its full intensity.

If one would form this habit by constant will power of keeping on smiling, being the soul of Release, by not taking sharp breaths or holding breaths, one would not stimulate the nerves that cause the heart excitement. This will permit the heart to rest a little longer between its beats.

Here is the "old secret" of releasing the heart by not exciting the heart, by not receiving the intensity of sensations that are coming to and from the brain. This is true in the thought kingdom also.

Hate, intense or otherwise; worry, severe or light; anxiety, little or great; fear, whether it be terror or only a slight apprehension; all these emotional thought processes are giving intense sensations to the body. As these sensations are passing through the back of the neck they are also exciting the heart.

At the very appearance of such a thought or emotion, suppose one took a slow deep breath and exhaled slowly. One would release the intense sensations by relaxing the receptor.

Suppose one learned to bring about a state of delightful smile at such an instance of thought. The severe sensations of hate, worry, anxiety, and kindred emotions would always diminish to such a point that one's brain and body would be relaxed, causing the sensation of life to be frail and delicate, and not clumsy, rough and tense.

This alone shall teach man to control his heart.

This calls for a new habit of life.

One has to train one's self to bring about this habit, or die.

The average person does not know how much of a "living dead" he is. It is not until his heart has received a definite damage by constantly interrupted and abrupt beatings, that he begins to feel the process of decay and death.

The training should be to teach this method to the children at school so that they would learn early not to live intensively but extensively. It would make a broadminded, released humanity of happiness and peace, orderly and law abiding, rather than chaotic and neurotic beings who live the life of civilized savages who do not know from one moment to the next whether they are "coming or going."

In this day and age when people are living sufficiently unto the headlines of newspapers; and sufficiently unto the yellings of radios and complexities of moving pictures; when life is nothing but one window shopping after another; and life is nothing but a succession of excitement and depression, depression and excitement; in waking or in sleeping; the science of medicine cannot keep pace with the possibilities of heart trouble and heart degeneration with all the medicines and heart treatments at its disposal.

The doctor is, and should be, the only active agent of nature and God with regard to the human body. And people who "violate" the laws of God and nature–the doctor is helpless to assist them when God fails.

The public, the spoiled neurotic, must not be flattered. But if anybody loved mankind, he would point out to them that they should learn to live sanely and calmly, without making the lives of themselves and others miserable, unhealthy and unsound by turning the day and night into a savage dance with tomahawks.

The Mechanism

Part I

Now we shall try to understand how the senses excite the heart, and how training of the same senses can relieve the heart. We shall study the mechanism.

The entire technique is Release of the receptor system.

The technique of heart control therefore would be a technique of Release of the receptor system in the brain (cerebrum).

The sense organs could be classified as follows:

1. The senses aroused by mechanical stimulation are touch, pain, muscle sense, equilibrium, and hearing.

2. The senses aroused by chemical stimulation are taste, smell, and the sensations of hunger, thirst, fatigue, nausea, etc.

3. The temperature sense.

4. The sense of sight stimulated by light.

5. The internal sense, that is, receptors inside the body such as muscle sense, equilibrium, pain, hunger, thirst, nausea, fatigue.

6. The external sense, that is receptors on the surfaces of the body which get information from the outside world. They are contact senses and projecting senses.

Now, if one does not bring about anxiety, pressure and tension to receive these sensations coming from these sources, one has automatically released the receptors.

The layman may easily learn this habit of not receiving sensations tensely, that is, without a tremendous amount of pressure.

The fight with gravity, for that is what it is, meeting friction by friction, is the beginning of heart excitement. Receiving sensations with release and a smile is the process of relaxation.

Here, we are giving you the final laws of life. Receive every sensation with the Release of the receptor center, with joy and happiness, and you will live a long, happy life. Receive the sensation with a grouch and lack of a sense of play and you begin to die slowly.

Receive the sensation, yea, all sensations, with a smile and lightness, with a sense of play and childish happiness, and you shall have released the receptors of sensations which generally excite you and your heart.

Part II

Now we shall study the mechanism more carefully and very patiently.

The medulla oblongata, in the back of the neck, is the center through which all nerve impulses must pass.

There are three nerve centers, like central stations of a telephone or telegraph system, located in this medulla oblongata.

1. The respiratory center, from which nerves (like telegraph or telephone wires) run to the muscles of the lungs, the chest cavity, and the diaphragm, and regulate the breathing of the individual.

(This has been shown at length for the layman in the section entitled "Breath Is Life.")

2. The vaso-constrictor center, from which nerves run to all parts of the body and cause the clamping or relaxing of the arteries, veins and blood vessels, thereby exciting or relaxing the internal organs, glands, muscles and tissues, etc. The general constriction or relaxation of the person greatly depends upon the system regulated from this center.

3. The cardiac center, from which the nerves running to the heart and also to the local center of the heart, called the cardiac plexus, regulate the slowness or fastness of the heart beat.

The heart is an independent animal.

It is perhaps a child of the sea. Perhaps it learned to beat incessantly from the mother sea. It has a long biological history. True to its nature, it learned to rise and fall like the tide and ebb of the sea.

It has been shown many times recently through inventions and discoveries that the heart can be taken out of the body and kept alive while the body may die. Its beats go on outside of the human body, showing that the nerves of the body alone do not cause its beats. It can go on beating alone without the interference of the nerves.

But the nerves of the body coming from the neck to a center in the chest cavity, called the cardiac plexus (plexus meaning a bundle of nerves and nerve fibers), do increase or diminish the excitement of these spontaneous beats of the heart.

The heart when it is absolutely left alone, and free from the interference of these nerve impulses, and so long as it can get its food and rest, will work rhythmically as an independent animal and rest between beats.

The four different parts of the heart, called the valves, do not work all at the same time. While one set is working, the other set is resting. In this way they are getting eight-hour shifts alternately as in a machine factory.

Almost mechanically, like the pistons of the motor of a car, they will go smoothly and nicely and automatically if they are only left alone and free of the impulses from the nerves.

Heart control, therefore, is control of these nerve impulses.

Therefore, let us talk about nerve control.

For the layman it is sufficient to know that a set of nerves, called the cardiac augmentory nerves, excites the heart. These nerves go to the back of the neck, the medulla oblongata, and when stimulated they excite the heart.

Then again, through the back of the neck and starting from the cranium of the brain (the tenth cranial nerve or vagus), there comes another set of nerves, called the cardiac inhibitory nerves, which goes to the heart plexus and also to the muscles of the heart. These nerves quiet down the beat of the heart.

It is this set of nerves that the doctors stimulate with the medicine digitalis to bring about the quieting of the heart, enough, so that the heart gets more rest between the beats.

Our task is to stimulate this cardiac inhibitory center. The center from which the nerves come, pass through the medulla oblongata and go inside the heart.

The methods of Yoga, therefore, would be such as to effect the inhibition of the heart by the stimulation of these cardiac inhibitory nerves.

There is another great task to be undertaken by us.

The heart when excited not only beats louder and faster, but the excitement caused by the nerves breaks up its rhythm. Jerky beats of the heart are more troublesome than fast beats of the heart.

We suggest a method whereby the average person may learn how to bring about smoothness in the heart beats which will keep up a beautiful dance of the heart, rather than a rough, jerky, chaotic, and mad beat of the heart, like an automobile going through a torn-up road.

This book therefore will do two things for the layman:

1. It will teach him how to give more rest to his heart.

2. In rest or in action his heart shall learn to beat with perfect mathematical rhythm and smoothness.

This is the heart control by Yoga.

Yoga Control

Again we find that heart control means control of the nerves exciting or inhibiting the heart beats.

Now let us proceed very slowly and see what causes the excitement of the cardiac augmentor center.

First, the incoming "muscle sense" from the muscles of the body going through the neck to the brain, stimulates this central station, called the augmentor center, and causes it to be excited.

It is very simple to see then, that as a person uses his muscles violently, his heart rate will be fast along with it. On the other hand, as a person sits down, lies down, or is quiet with his muscles, the inhibitory center will be stimulated and the impulses will be checked, thus causing the heart to beat slower.

Is this not very simple to understand even for a child?

Now we see, when we are walking automatically, the heart is not violently excited. When we are working automatically, when all our actions and thoughts are falling into a rhythmic dance, the heart is not going in jerks or beating violently.

It is also clear, even for a child to understand, that it is the violent, sudden, and abrupt, jerky moves of muscular activity and the muscle sense which are the source of all the trouble.

Here is the beginning of the Death of the Heart.

Then again, as with the "muscle sense," so also with the brain cells and brain fibers in the brain. As jerky thoughts and abrupt and sudden thoughts spurt out in the brain, with fits of emotions, they pass through the same center in the back of the neck and stimulate the augmentor center so that it gets excited, and through the augmentor nerve impulses causes the heart to beat faster.

Please, please read this very carefully.

Now, you get an idea. Instantly, with a violent intake of breath you start a process of thoughts. Here is the jerky, sharp constriction, and here is the sudden excitement of the heart.

Could you not have started your precious idea or precious thought with a little slow rhythm. With a sense of play, release and a smile?

Was the life and death of the nation or of the whole world at stake that you started your idea in your brain with such an explosion and jerk?

No, your only excuse is habit.

Your habits therefore will kill you unless you change them.

We shall, therefore, suggest a method, with your consent and your understanding and your sympathy, whereby we shall understand how to bring about a soft rhythm in the beats of the heart so that life will go on happily and peacefully, without the fear of decay and death.

Yoga Control Instrument

Here is the revelation.

If you *can only learn* to live in the *realm of feeling* instead of thinking, you will have learned the secret.

Every time an idea is in your brain, and every time you are thinking, you are sending out motor impulses, that is, a tendency to action and activity of the muscles; for you cannot act without the help of the muscles.

But, along with that, there is a sensory sensation going on in the body and the brain.

Suppose you learn to feel this sensory sensation as you feel the taste of an apple or a lump of sugar. Immediately this feeling will take your mind into the realm of perception which will diminish the heart rate.

Now, if these sensations which are coming to the brain are increased, your heart beats will increase. But the moment *your mind begins to feel* the sensations that are coming to the brain, meaning pain, pleasure, sensual or sensuous thrills—when you are busy *feeling* them, there will be calmness of the heart. And when you let these sensations become your master and drive your mind crazy, your heart will also go crazy along with it.

Mind therefore is not you.

You are the life. You are the sensation. You are the feeling, and your mind is the shadow, the leftover of you. Mind tries. You become it.

You cannot control the heart or the mind by mind, meaning thoughts. The more you will try to control them, the more you will excite the heart and the head.

All these exercises will help you to get rid of your mind, and show you that there is a you in you which is your soul.

We are not talking religion, metaphysics, or sentimentalism, but we are talking a definite science.

First of all, you yourself are in the *sensory aspect of life* and not the *motor aspect.*

We have pointed out in an article in *Yogas* how people suffer and die through motor degeneration of the body and the mind. In the same *Yogas* we have pointed out, how motor regeneration of the nerves is effected through our method of quieting down the heart, or hibernation of the body by the process of Samadhi.

In all the exercises you take, the aim would be first to find out how you yourself will effect a quieting of your body and mind by these exercises. And when you have found the method of quieting, it is up to you to create the new habit.

All the exercises will show you that you can quiet down by giving up the muscular exertions or volition with which you excite the muscles. You and not your mind.

Of course you will learn them when you are quiet. But your work will be to keep up these quiet attitudes during work, action and thought. That is the hardest thing to do. And yet, unless you do it, there is no doctor in the world who can calm down your heart, and save you from possible heart trouble, and heart degeneration, if you go on with your old habits of life.

You will find that excitement of the heart is always identified with excitement of the lungs and constriction of the muscles and nerves. You will also find that quieting of the heart means also the quieting of the lungs, and relaxation of the muscles.

Therefore the way to bring enjoyment and happiness in the muscle sense, is to feel your body and the muscles and the nerves as you would feel a lump of sugar in your mouth, and the hard work will be easy. Your fatigue will vanish and you will know a new type of happiness.

Automatically a new life will dawn in you.

Of course the habits of your old life, the ghosts of your past, will always try to drag you back into the life of old constrictions and sufferings.

To make it worse, not only your own habits but the whole world of ideas along with all the ideas you get from your friends, books, newspapers, radios, and what not – all of them will conspire to bring you back into the old life.

And the most pitiful aspect of it all is that those who try to teach you to take care of your body and mind will give you such ideas which will cause more constriction, more excitement and more heart trouble. *They will not leave you alone.*

And you will not let your heart alone, and your heart will not leave the rest of the body alone.

Therefore it calls for the whip. The whip is the will to will and keep on willing.

Will is not a prize fighter. It starts with saying "No" to volition and effort–the hardest thing in the world.

Will rises with a smile from the feeling side of life.

Yoga Control of Glands

Now we are going to tell you another interesting story which is the story of the real cause of your heart trouble, apart from the muscles of the body and their violent exertions which cause your heart trouble.

On both sides of the top of the kidneys there are two little glands called suprarenals or adrenals. They secrete a hormone, just one part of which mixed with four hundred million (1 to 400,000,000) parts of water is sufficient to give tone to the muscles of the body and keep up the sense of well-being throughout the body and the mind.

This adrenal secretion is poured into the blood and the blood distributes it everywhere in the body.

Now, as any emotion rises in the brain, such as hate, anger, worry, fear, anxiety, and all their relatives, these glands pour more juice into the blood. Along with this juice of the adrenals, whenever this condition arises in the body, the thyroids from near the throat pour their juice, further exciting the whole bodily activity.

And whenever the adrenals pour their juice into the blood, another little gland in the brain called the pituitary gland, pours its little juice. These three together, along with other glands, cause havoc in the body and the mind.

So when one is under the storm of these juices, one cannot easily stop and be calm in a second.

Were it possible to show you the picture of a human being, even when he is praying in a "Billy Sunday" meeting, you would see a picture of a chaotic, electrical storm inside his brain. At that time you might easily see what is happening to the heart due to these physical processes.

When a person hates somebody, he is only hurting himself by killing his own heart. When one is inflamed with a sense of injustice done to him, his country, or his race (right or wrong), through the process of vengeance and anger, he is killing his own heart.

When one is despising and loathing things that seem immoral or unethical, he is not pleasing God but he is killing his own heart.

When you see ladies and gentlemen "sticking up their nose" at things, we know that they are killing themselves by creating a venom secretion in their body, a cell secretion which we have called "Hala-Hal" in our book *A Strange Language*.

In all these violent emotional processes even in so-called good emotions, such as tremendous excitement of joy and hope, the heart beats are going on in jerks and violence, not only through muscular tension but also through the pouring of the juices of these glands into the blood stream.

More than that, all the unsatisfied and unsated hopes of the body and the mind cause violent excitations and desires. And when these remain unsatisfied they give pangs to the heart through mental tortures.

More people die of heart trouble and have their hopes blasted mercilessly in this dear age of artificial appetites and artificial satisfactions.

We are writing with love for humanity. Therefore, we have to strip man's mind of the sham and hypocrisy with which he has cloaked himself in the black cloak of death.

Love dictates that we tell him the nude truth although it may shock his ethical knowledge of the past.

The young boys and girls in their courtship days are continually exciting their passion of sex impulses with violent hopes of the body and glands which are arousing the heart beats, too. But when they come home they feel depression of the heart through sex despair.

Heaven only knows to what extent the heart trouble of the younger generation is due to the system of "courting the ship," called courtship. Nor does the story end here. The entire mixing of sexes during the day and night is repeating the story ad infinitum. One may easily imagine the onslaught of emotional pressure that is being brought upon the heart.

Then we have economic arousals and depressions due to the attacks of vanity. The desire to be brilliant, clever and outshining in the eyes of friends and the public is sufficient to cause any heart to undergo volcanic actions and depthless depressions.

Looking at God's man, one would ask where does the normalcy of this man start, and where does it end?

To him, therefore, we shall plead the quieting of the adrenal, thyroid, pituitary and other glands. In other words, we shall plead for the quieting of his blood.

When the blood is hot, the heart is burning. When the blood is cool, the soul of the man is cool also.

It is the coolness of the body and the mind which alone will take care of the heart. Coolness therefore is heart control.

Only one thing will control glands. And instantly. Do it, and find out.

Surrender to life with an unreserved childish and playful smile and say : "Thy Will be done."

Dreams of Heart

As we unbind the scroll of this little prayer, we are merely dreaming of a thousand years hence when people will be born with flower hearts. People who will be so happy within that they will see only beauty without.

Today, critics will spit on these pages. Tomorrow free men and women will salvage them from the archives of neglect and read them with a fondness for this pen.

For we have dived depth below depth into the deep of man's heart and found hushed founts of freedom, happiness and power that will explode into a thousand fragrant flowers some day. It is this heredity of the heart that man shall bequeath unto the hearts of posterity.

True it is—today, hearts are stifled by the fumes of venom, and are smitten down by the lightnings from some ruthless and heartless clouds, bleeding beneath the trampling feet of the haughty rulers of man—

True it is—today, the terror stricken hearts of the earth even dare not whisper a note of hope to other hearts in despair lest their drumbeats and bugle call strangle the very pulsation of the heart—

True it is—today, all hearts must stifle their desolate sobs in the depth of night lest the very breeze betray the existence of hearts to the wrath of the victors among men—

Yet, somehow, we know, there will be peace on earth again willed by the sovereign of peace.

Again shall the silver rivers of the spring come dancing down the hillsides, dishevelled in the silver white of the moon. And again, shall the unnamed, arched lilies come floating on the blue and white crests of the laughing waves of the streams—

Again shall strange strains of some honied distant symphony, mingled shades and lights of a myriad tones, like an outpour of a million rainbows in one, come floating down from some distant land enthralling the very light of the day—as shall the bridal breeze melt on the green leaves of the trees in sweet languor of tremulous June—

Again, the mornings, noon and dusk shall be mellow on the shores of light—as shall for long hours of long days all young lives bask in the fragile honey of the sun—

Life shall be a song again—

An unending song of eternity of love.

And one crooning, white night of the moon while all eyes on earth shall be closed in the silken sleep of bashful dreams, an unknown bird from some unknown heaven shall pour forth its undying melody across the unending azure—

And my own heart shall leap out from the deep within me and soar away with the strain of its aerial loveliness, to the land of the stars.

For morrow shall dawn with a new light in the heaven of my man.

And then, then alone, I shall make all bold to assert Hearts shall smile again.

The immortal heart of man.

And then, then alone

Hearts shall tell the beads...

This precious Heart—

It shall be the throne of my Master.

INTERNAL RESPIRATION

INTRODUCTION TO PART THREE

Our final prayer is that Love may so dawn in your consciousness, bloom in your life that this Light may envelop you as you in turn give out to others—not scolding them but giving soul to them. They can't see the Light until the Flash appears in the Sky and changes the brain.

Before this happens, there will be many tribulations, volcanic eruptions, the terrestrial atmosphere of our everyday life will change, what with poisonous vapors, virus chemicals, and at last—a Famine of Breath—

Only those who know *how to breathe* will survive.

Pundit Acharya

I.

HOW TO REVIVE THIS LOST FACULTY

The moment we talk about breathing, we think of human or animal breathing in terms of external respiration.

There is no need of repeating information you can gather elsewhere from any university. Rather I am calling attention to some of the facts you may have had in the past. Also, I am suggesting certain things to you from the applied side. To laymen, the application is more important than the theory.

Mistakes of Ordinary Breathing

We shall see the mistakes first of ordinary breathing.

Breathing is an automatic thing with human beings—a nervous thing. A set of nerves excites the diaphragm, the diaphragm exciting another set of nerves and muscles, which causes the deflation of the diaphragm, and the breathing therefore is a result of this play of the diaphragm. The muscles concerned are the abdominal muscles and intercostal muscles—not the chest muscles but the alveoli or lung muscles, etc.

The reason for breathing is to give oxygen to the bloodstream, so that the bloodstream can carry it to the rest of the body. This oxygen is an important element.

All this is information but the thing important to us would be to know how we have degenerated from the *trend of evolution*—how, possibly, we have degenerated from the rest of the evolutionary path by the change that we have made.

Our external respiration is a great change from the rest of the animal kingdom. Here we see an animal going under the sand and staying for two years without breathing in our sense. Even when the apparatus of external breathing has appeared in the scale of evolution, even then the animal could go and hibernate for two years.

You see the beginning of the Yogi. What one animal could do, another animal could do. It is possible. Yoga has become news to the western world. It is not news. It is a biological affair. It is not an innovation but a revival of the thing that was already there.

Nose and mouth are not a necessity–not a need, but a luxury, and this luxury we have misused so much that, like a rich man's child, we are so spoiled we cannot do without.

Objective of Breathing

The objective of breathing is internal respiration and not external respiration: the *use* of the oxygen in the exchange. This dependence on the nose first, and secondly on the mouth for the respiration is something man has developed by loss of something else that is very vital. The organism had known something which it has lost or blunted in the nose and mouth breathing.

I am inclined to think the heart came first in the process of evolution rather than the lungs. Whether it did or not, we are sure that in the vegetable kingdom, the lungs have not as yet appeared and still the plants undergo the process of respiration. All that we mean by respiration is the *exchange of oxygen and carbon dioxide.* The need for carbon dioxide and oxygen is just as important to the plant kingdom as the animal kingdom.

Plants Ingest Air–Why Can't Man?

Let us plunge at once into the plant kingdom which had a suction power in order to draw the nutrition directly. Who knows but what man had the same avenue of ingesting water from the ground with his bare feet and bare body, sucking in the vitamins of sunlight from the sun, oxygen from the compound of earth, and ingesting air by straining it!

The capillaries in man are no longer capable of the action of the alveoli—they are so blunt. There was a time when the capillaries used to work directly to take the oxygen. Man with other higher organs has completely lost that function in the process of specialization.

Now it happens that a man cannot possibly live without breathing through his nose. If anything happens to his external apparatus, he is done for. In asthma particularly, we see what he has done by giving up his internal processes and creating an artificial process externally. To me external respiration is *artificial*.

Do you not see the thought processes of man are bound up with his respiration? He is so mixed up with the visual process that *he cannot think without eyes*. Now we know that man cannot think without his respiration. Watch it. Try to think without interfering with your respiration. As emotions vary, your respirations vary.

As the spatiality of your thought processes becomes smaller, breathing is harder. As they occupy more space, become extensive, it becomes easier. You cannot dissociate your breathing process. You are continually breathing bodily, and since the blood has to come to the heart, your heart process is involved in it. Now you see why the arteriosclerosis, why the heart trouble.

Biologically we shall proceed and see what man is doing. Man doesn't possibly believe he could take oxygen through any other organ except through his nose and mouth.

See the trees and plants. We see that they have to have *cellular* effort to suck air as we do through nose and mouth.

We have not changed with the mouth or the throat. We still have to pull the air from outside to inside through the nose. This is a muscular effort—a nervous effort. Nerves are concerned and muscles obey. It is a chemical process of releasing the h-ion, exciting the phrenic nerve, working the diaphragm, etc.

I remind you, this pull through the nose is a specialization, a luxury. The intercostal muscles are the ones concerned. These muscles are doing the job dictated by the nerves.

Why couldn't the same nerves ask the other voluntary muscles of the body to take a share in the pull and relieve the nose of this work? In asthma and sinus trouble, you would not suffer so much.

You saw what the lower animals could do without breathing through the nose. Now you see how the Yogis have not found anything new but have revived something that was lost. I am not giving information but I am suggesting something very practical.

You have seen, by indulging in this luxury of breathing through special organs, how we have degenerated. Since we mix our thoughts with our breathing process, we actually cause tension in certain parts of the body where relaxation is necessary. How much disturbance of the viscera is dependent upon bad breathing and nose breathing alone, is a study in itself.

Experiment and Find Out

This is a scientific work. Let us do some laboratory work and find out. Suppose we say: *"For the time being, I am going to cut short my breathing. I will make it very shallow."*

Open your mouth and be very calm and gentle. Don't try to breathe. Notice the anxiety! As though you won't live! With the push of resistance is coming the impatience.

See how easily and peacefully you get along breathing as shallow as humanly possible. You are still living and your physiological processes are going on very nicely. You have attained relaxation without the laziness of relaxation.

The thermal sense will show your temperature inside is rising as you shut up this breathing. See also how your entire glandular system will be quieted—thyroid, adrenal, and all the related glands—by cutting out this anxiety neurosis called external breathing.

Just a shallow breath—hardly any breath—then rest.

Suppose you form the habit. As you go about your job and are thinking, begin to free yourself from this external respiration by the nose in shallow breathing. It is not that you are not using the oxygen. You are making full use of the oxygen instead of the oxygen begging the cells: "Please take me."

Some day a great bio-physician shall show that *death equals the decline of the osmotic pressure,* meaning the food and oxygen go begging in the bloodstream and the cells do not take it. So much attention has been paid to the food and oxygen from outside that no one pays attention to the cells themselves.

You cannot mechanically excite the cells as you excite the central nervous system, and the nerves will not allow the cells to do anything without paying tax to the nervous system. There are sixty-three thousand miles of blood vessels, and wherever there are blood vessels, there are governmental systems to dictate to them—the nerves. Not psychologically will you change them, as this will not reach into the habits which have been interfering with the tissues and blood vessels.

Why look at the last result: arteriosclerosis, the slackening of the walls? There was a time when there was no central nervous system, when there were no nerves. To man it is news: flesh without nerves. But we are still that protoplasm. We are not subject to nerves as much as we think.

If we could *vitalize this protoplasm to suck in food and nutrition and air* (let me call it air instead of oxygen) *once more as we did in the tree days and in the lower-vertebrate days,* if we could do that, we shall have stopped the tension in the tissue realm and in the vascular realm.

Retraining the Nerves

The children of medicine will look at the mental tension. There is no such thing as mental tension. There is only nerve tension. If we retrain the nerves to recreate the suction to pull in the air as the nose does, we shall begin to recharge our battery more fully, and we shall know *real* relaxation.

I told you to cut down your breathing. As you climb stairs, instead of fighting with your breath (the pull of the earth vs. your abdomen)—the unused muscles of the abdomen are so lazy that the diaphragm cannot do the work and you have shortness of breath—at that time, *don't breathe.* See what does happen.

A coordination would take place between the belly and the

stairs. You are becoming a free man. Free not from gravity but free from your nerves. Minus that fight. Man's greatest fight is with nerves, his sensory nerve endings and his motor nerve endings which have made a wreck out of him finally.

Man cannot feel the subtle touches of air pressure, and other things present in the atmosphere. The animals can. This subtle perception was lost because of specialization. This specialization took place because man is the only animal who has power of deduction and other mental processes. He has abused this privilege by using the luxury of nose breathing and made a monkey out of himself.

Your objective is not economic or political freedom, but freedom from your sympathetic adrenal system. You are not a serf of your wants. You will experience this when you free yourself from breathing: your external respiration. You will fully understand these things when you go back to the tree days and with your hands and your bare feet *pull in the air with your whole body.*

You are beginning to see how you revive your body. You are no longer tense nervously. The constriction of the blood vessels is not taking place.

I will not promise in advance, in case of arteriosclerosis, that you will regenerate the arteriosclerosis, but this will keep well people well. Those who are sincere know it is the greatest thing in life to remain well. You cannot do it by good intentions but by good habits. The habits I refer to are physiological and not mental. Mental habits are to fool with.

Physiological Habits Important

How you sit, how you walk, how you get up from the bed, what you do in bed, these are the physiological habits. Instead of taking laxatives, what you do in the bathroom is important. If you injure the nerves innervating the colon, what can you expect? If you have trained yourself to have a certain number of evacuations a day, how can you expect, the moment this is disturbed and you are taking a drug or something else to do the work, that the colon will behave properly? Through your nerve pathway, you have spoiled that colon.

You are alarmed by the increasing child delinquency. How about your colon? Making "one world" and "brotherhood" is not the problem. The real problem is your colon, your constipation. Not once has it been taught that you are responsible for your colon, this spoiled brat of yours.

Have you ever known colon breathing? If suction of air and water can go through one hole, can't it go through another hole? Do you know that parts of the colon remain voluntary muscles? But of course you will have to have a special gadget with all kinds of paraphernalia and perfume to pet that colon with some water inside.

Your colon is not to be ashamed of. No organ is vulgar. That which gives you life is a holy animal. As a quadruped you used to jar it by moving the hind leg. Now you take a fashionable walk on Broadway talking about Wall Street. And the colon talks about Wall Street too. It waits for the fashionable medicine. Can't you see the inference?

This man cannot go on living like that for long. The therapies and medicines are becoming so gigantic that every man, woman and child is a living therapy. But no one calls attention to the man himself who will not control his colon. This is true of his stomach too and above all his respiration.

Reviving Our Lost Faculties

After awhile we shall learn to go to the canal where the food goes, and stir up activity there.

Suppose *we begin to breathe out.* Gradually we excite the cells. The nerves do not like it, but gradually we will have control.

Forget books and *begin to pull your body. Then begin to inhale through the whole body* instead of that little effort you have been making.

You will see breathing is not the internal respiration we talk about. Use that oxygen which is two-thirds heat and one-third motion instead of always complaining to the landlord for heat. Heat yourself. Lazy people will not generate any heat inside and the external heat from the radiator kills people. If anything kills, it is this artificial heat and light.

Translate that light into sound and you could go crazy with the noise. Thank God, Nature has tremendous power of resistance. Otherwise you would be stark mad from light alone.

In the midst of all this artificiality, we learn to revive ourselves, our lost heritage—as the trees. The same with water and the earth. You will perform a bath or shower. The shower cleanses the dirt outside but it does not cleanse the dirt within. You are water—I am forced to say these things to you over and over again—two-thirds of your bones are earthy matter. You are dirt, you are minerals. That's your bones. So you cannot get free from dirt. And you can't get free from salt water. You came from the sea, from the ocean. So commune with the water when you are bathing.

Your nerves will not permit. They will shut up the receptor system. The Brahmins sit in water and cleanse inside. This means not bathing but mixing with water. When you are in the water there, *suck it in.* You are water. Isn't that a beautiful thing to believe? I am water, air, heat, full of electricity (inside and outside of me) to be used as a play. People come to the country to get it. It's inside of you all the time.

You are a bundle of constricted nerves whose result is arteriosclerosis at last. It is high time you change by reviving some of the faculties you had from the beginning.

Calm down. How? Count sheep? No.

Shut up your nose breathing, open your mouth, and relax. Make your breathing shallower and shallower, and the rate of exchange is becoming slower and slower. An internal hibernation is taking place. You cannot think "Coney Island." No circus. Your breathing almost comes to nil slowly.

First you will get sleepy. Have a talk with yourself. You have never slept. You have never known the sweetness of sleep because you have gone to bed taking the human society in your arms and lived with it in your bed. "What did he say about me?" In between the devil gets hold of you and puts you through knotholes we call sleep. So long as you go through the process, you think it's all right.

Security of Animal Foothold

You have never known life, have never known animal eating, animal sleeping, animal defecation, animal relaxation, and animal foothold. This creature has a foothold. Everything has a foothold on earth. Man hasn't. Every time the doorbell rings, he is scared. Unless he makes so much a week or a month, he is scared. He is bragging to himself. Economic security is not his trouble. He is afraid of himself.

"Can I have any respect for myself? I am Ph.D., D.D., Litt.D., M.D. . . . Suppose I sit on the floor? I am a gentleman or a lady. If a bill collector came to see me, he would say I am crazy." Unless a man is fully dressed, he is a bum.

This is an artificial want we have built up in our brain, our intellect. We shall be free from it. Gather things, come to any deduction you like, but live like an animal. You do it anyway secretly. So do it publicly.

First security is breath. Revolt against it. Open your mouth. *Breathe through the mouth.* You will say: Dust will get in there, germs will get in there. If you breathe through the mouth, suppose germs do get in there. The mouth is full of germs anyway.

In high blood pressure, arterial pressure, *breathe through the mouth.* Cut out this fight with the nose.

In heart cases, digitalis is given. You will give the tenth cranial nerve release by cutting down the breath. As soon as you feel sleepy, breathing would be hard again. Peace is peace from this voluntary exchange.

What happens? Internal respiration takes place. The exchange takes place normally inside. There is a balance between the two which is peace. It is a chemistry. Mind is only the result of it. The only thing mind can do about it is the attitude which will change. Mind can institute that change of attitude.

I repeat, *infinitely slowly, gently,* (when you become gentle, there's a chance for the involuntary muscles to wake up), *slowly cause an inner pull, an inner suction and begin to feel your muscles inwardly.* I think I told you, you wouldn't believe it, that you can at last feel your viscera by the nerve-awakening inside. This will give you freedom from tension, and then your glands, your pancreas can function.

It is not what you have eaten but what you have done after eating. You have "raised Cain" with yourself and you blame your food. You haven't allowed the glands of the stomach and intestines to do their work. While eating you are busy freeing the small nations. You don't know what you ate. The mouth ate but the cells did not eat. You socialized and settled all the problems of the community, but they did not eat. A dog and cat would ask you: When you eat, why don't you eat? The animal is co-conscious.

The Co-conscious Man

I predict that in the twenty-first or fiftieth century men will be born who will be co-conscious and responsible for themselves. When they say I, they will mean I, the master. They will be ashamed to talk about their stomach, their glands, and other organs. Because it is they who have allowed their lazy organs inside to behave that way.

Teachers will learn first and then students.

One of the greatest disturbers of respiration is your talk. There are three kinds of talk. One is to get real information which is needed. The second is flirting, coquetry, salesmanship by which you get food, vanity, or sex, one of the three hungers. There's . another kind of talk in which you show how stupid the other fellow is—the one who is talked to. You drown him with your language, vanquish him with nouns, adjectives and verbs.

When you talk, ask yourself: "Am I giving any information? Is this necessary or coquetry?" Coquetry is a broad subject—to sell something or to create scandal. The third talk is to train the other fellow, shut him up, don't give him a chance. In this process, ask yourself: "How many calories do I need to do this talking? Where does this energy come from?"

A charming young man asked me: "How is it I am impotent at this age? I do not have any organic trouble."

When I said: "You have just so much energy for your work, and whatever little energy you have left goes out through your mouth—what energy would you have left?" he said: "What shall I do?"

I said: "Shut up. Learn silence."

Therapy of Silence

Now I come from a very ignorant class of people in India who have for ages preached silence and in the western world, the time is coming when it will know people of silence. Silence does not mean shutting up your lips, but inner relaxation, a dilation, a mixing with this thing that's going on there. The human nitwit cannot see how much space there is there.

Get drunk on this space inside there. It will calm down your central nervous system. It will give you such education that no man could ever talk to you. Infinite space. Air, sunshine, moonlight, storm and rain. Freedom from talking to other people. Nobody to please and nobody's got to please you.

The greatest disease from the moment I am awake is I have to entertain somebody. If no one is around, a cat or a dog. I am telling you a shortcut. Watch your breathing at that moment. Throw the newspaper away. *"Here I go. I won't breathe."* Then mix with space. Suppose you are so many years old. Then it is high time to try something new.

"I am wasting time today, I had better breathe fast and get somewhere"—old habits. The time is coming when people will experiment with a new method of life and not look for therapy.

There is a new posture therapy. Nerves cannot be trained by new postures.

I say this in all sincerity because there is a dire need in the United States, and other countries follow the United States. The nerve diseases are increasing so much that they are desperately thinking of new therapies. Every day they invent a new therapy. Somebody writes another volume of Latin or Greek jawbreaking words, and the patients become crazier and crazier. When Freud's book came out, every cat, dog and bedbug took up Freud, this new psychology as a vogue. They will give you a dose of psychology. Every psychologist needs a psychologist.

Gentleness and Will

We have a marvelous instrument known as Will. Will is silent. Will is determination. Will can do miracles but this Will cannot work with our emotions. This Will is not a motor activity. It is very sweet. It is a reflection of our continued existence. It knows.

If I say: "I am going to do this tomorrow," my Will says: "You know you are a liar—you are not going to do it at that time." Will does not make rash promises.

Will says: "I give myself to You, all that I am, my hands, my feet, my eyes, my mouth, my language, my thoughts, my incarnation, all that I could possibly be, all that I dream of being, I give at once to You. Change me now." This humility is prayer, a Will that can come only from within.

It's in your system. If it doesn't awake, wait. On your deathbed, it may come. It will come. This change takes place. Then you will begin to know what I am talking about. That gives you a gentleness, a foothold. That gives a sweet condition in the body.

When a man or woman like that comes to the hospital, the patients feel better. One man like that in the town, the town feels better. One man of humility. One "gentle" man.

Gentleness is the least breath. Gentleness does not require a lot of puffing. *"Thy Will be done."* A very simple fact. Understand what it means, *"Thy* Will." The Will that I have is Thy Will, not my Will. It only works through my brain.

This knowledge, this wisdom your university cannot give. This is immortality. You don't die after that. Then you begin to fall into the organic realm. Free from the nerves.

II.

HOW TO VITALIZE THE PROTOPLASM

For the well-being of body and mind, more important than food is energizing the body.

You have to be absolutely loyal to the law. Otherwise you will be dizzy and have nausea.

The law is play. You have to play like a child. With a sense of humor. This will bring lightness.

As you are taking the exercises, if you forget that lightness, immediately you will get exhausted, and also you will feel a little nausea to start with. Then when you get used to it, the method will work.

These exercises will help elimination, assist you in throwing out the poisons. No matter how cold it is outside, you will sweat. When you have learned to sweat, you will know how to be clean.

The danger in the beginning is constriction, tightness, and then exhaustion. This would be because you are hurrying. If you have ever known what slowness is, now is the time to practice it. Then, you have to play.

Energizing the Body

Always start by drinking a glass of water first.

1.

First, you will sit straight. You have to sit straight. Otherwise, you won't be able to feel it. *Then sag the jaw.*

2.

Slowly, very slowly, take a breath. By slow we mean the air must be felt as thin. The air will not be thin unless you are light yourself and you are smiling inside. If I take a quick breath, I find it is thick, but as I *breathe slowly and smile*, it is thin.

You will not be able to breathe deeply until you learn exhalation. It is exhalation—throwing out the carbon dioxide from the body—rather than inhalation that is important. (Inside the body, all the cells and glands between the pelvis and the throat have every chemistry that the doctor can give. All medicines, if they are analyzed, become ions—carbon, hydrogen, oxygen, nitrogen, etc.) You will stir them up, make them work.

The liver is miraculous. It generates all kinds of antidotes to the poisons in the body. It's a regular chemical factory. As soon as a pathological condition exists, and germs get into the body, the cells themselves generate immunity—a secretion which makes one immune to the disease. The antidote is always there in the body but it generates at that time.

Science is finding that the body has all the medicines, but we must learn to stir them up. It takes a long, long time to learn.

3.
Start very slowly and laughingly. As you breathe out, feel the muscles in the chest cavity, the abdominal cavity, and all the muscles back and front. Slowly, smilingly, gently.

4.
Do this two or three times, then rest. Play, play, play. Make it more light, please, more thin. If there is any gas there, it will be stirred up. Take the navel (umbilicus) in.

5.
Touch and get the sensation from all the volitional muscles first.
Gradually you will be able to feel all the so-called involuntary muscles also, your stomach organs, everything.

6.
Play with the breath. Move the muscles and feel them as you breathe. Keep the heart calm. As long as you smile and laugh, the heart will remain calm.

This breathing will help to eliminate colds, sinus and throat troubles.

Drink a lot of water, then begin to breathe deeply as above. Peristaltic action will start immediately. Begin to *move* inside the body. Then gradually you will have a snake movement throughout and at last you will be able to get inside the chest, shoulders and throat cavities—*feeling the movement* of the breath there. *Bring the movement from the back, feel it in the back also.*

7.

As you breathe in air very softly, pull the air in from your hands. Inhale and exhale through the hands.

8.

Now pull the air in from the feet. Inhale and exhale through the feet and hands. You will feel the pull through all the nerves of the body. There are innumerable little arteries which you are working this way.

9.

As you are breathing like that, feel your muscles, particularly the back muscles, and exhale from the back. Oxidation then takes place there.

Cell oxidation-electrical sparks are generated. (See the "Laws of Oxidation" in "Breath Is Life," also "Delicate Mechanism of Feeding" in the same section for an understanding of how we feed the blood vessels with this oxygen carried by the lymph fluid.) Read these chapters over and over again and then come back to these exercises.

"At last my body is becoming my own. I am the master of my body and I can go anywhere in the body and control it."

How will you know you are there? By the sensation. Not mentally. You have got to get the practical sensation there; otherwise it is a ghost story.

10.

As you are breathing like that, feel your muscles. As you breathe and feel there, the cells there are getting their oxygen.

11.

The next step is: very gently and very smilingly, now get the same feeling only in rhythm. That's how you will sweat and go deeper and deeper. *Can you feel the stomach, the intercostal muscles, everything? Stir them up.* That's how we rejuvenate and keep eternal youth. It's just like an electric current going through the body, shiver after shiver.

Then we learn gradually to go up through the body. As we breathe pleasantly, we go up. (But a lazy body won't do it.) Then deeper and deeper. (This gives you just a glimpse of how the Yogis control their bodies.)

It can't be done by mind. Only by practice and absolute obedience to the law. Otherwise it's hallucination. The mind will not leave the body alone and that's how it becomes exhausted.

The earth is moving, going around, all the planets are moving, not exactly around, but sort of an ellipse formation. But there is a rhythm in it, a wave. There is attraction and repulsion going on. All occult waves, all ether waves are that.

12.

Now, bring that feeling in this wave. As you are breathing in and out, you bring a wave of that, and the wave goes through the inside of the body. As though you were drunk. It's a pleasant sensation.

13.

First, go into the wave. Then you will know what it feels like. You cannot know the water by thinking about it. You have to go into the water.

Thereby you are training all the brain cells gradually. If you do it from the head, then you will get dizzy. But you must do it from the body with the breath.

14.

Make the air very thin and light. Smilingly. The wave is felt with the air. You do not move the body.

15.

Now let the head go into it too. Then get that pleasant sensation the same as in swimming–a slight drunkenness.

The body becomes very light. You are living a different life from other people. Your magnetism is increasing, and if you do not bring a selfish wish at that time, you are powerful. You cannot get angry at such a time. There's too much good feeling inside. When you go in the street, you will find everything looks beautiful. Everything is changed. Gradually your eyes, face, everything will change—a softer look will come.

If you neglect any part of the body, that's where the disease will set in.

At such a time you cannot think. You are enjoying it.

16.

If you feel tightness in the neck, dissolve the neck. Let go of the tightness there. *Open the mouth as in wonder and loosen the jaw muscles.*

Bring that state of lightness when you are sitting down there. Don't look for an object. Now, in this light stage, almost a stupor, in this delightful so-called drunken stage, you will find that gradually a new light dawns. You are illuminated. The first stage of that will be that all the sensory nerves will tingle—in your flesh there will be a tingling going on, a delightful tingling.

17.

Practice it two or three times a day, but not too much at a time.

Anandum in Sanskrit is not joy, not pleasure therefore, but this peculiar nectar, joy which no one can show through words. A drunken joy but very ethereal inside the body and mind. Complete. It doesn't want anything. Everything is fulfilled. All other joy wants something.

Now you see what your oxygen is. This is the hormone of Amiya (see *A Strange Language* for understanding of Amiya). This is Amiya, the nectar which is in everything, in plants, animals, trees, mountains, rivers, every being and every cell of the universe.

From time to time human beings get a thrill but they don't know how to hold on to it. This is the thrill.

18.

Do you get the shivers now? The action current goes all over the body. If you are not getting the shivers, you are not giving up. You must surrender. There you go. . . . *Take this breath. You are giving yourself up in love's arms. You are safe. Nothing can hurt you.*

19.

Here it goes. Slowly you give up. You will feel all over the body these little pricks of energy, a peculiar heat.

Notice further you have forgotten how much you weigh. The weight has vanished. There is no more weight. It is sublimated. If you have learned that, you have made great progress.

20.

Morning time and night time, slowly, slowly travel all over the body and feel that pleasantness. Bless the whole body inside.

The day you have learned the difference between feeling and imagination, you have a key in your hand: the key to the door of a new world. That will be the day you find out the difference between seeing it or imagining it and *feeling* it. (Once the brain gets it, it won't admit that the body gets it.)

As you give up, unconsciously without knowing, you are giving up your awareness. That part of the brain that becomes aware is going to sleep, is getting drunk. What's actually happening is they are getting so much food there in those cells, they are gathering up their dendrons and going to sleep so the other part of the brain can wake up and go to work.

Consciousness is things—"motor tendencies" as Wundt stated—but this is not that consciousness. This is an awareness which has no dimensions, no space, time, solid, liquid or gas. It is lightless. It has no light or shadow. If you watch it, it won't be there. Watching is the negative or expression part. Energy is the other thing. We generate with the energy. We can't generate when watching.

21.

If you begin to watch there, you will get into an astral whirlpool, see all kinds of colors and other things. *When that happens, give up that temptation. Feel the sensation.* Do not watch it.

Earthly temptations cannot be given up by repression. The more we try to repress, the more desire there is.

22.

Therefore, you don't try to repress the temptation. You just bring more

of the positive into it. The more feeling you bring, the more it drops away.
"Lead me not into temptation." We don't ask for strength to fight
temptation, but *"Don't lead me to it at all."* Do you see the
difference? He Who knew said: "Lead me not into temptation."
You don't even meet the temptation. You are busy somewhere
else. Automatically you are not led to temptation.

Now, when you are so happy, if someone says: "Will you have a
glass of Scotch?" you will say: "I have something better than
Scotch here. It's a delightful thing I've got here. I've outgrown
that." If you practice this kind of breathing, your whole body will
be purified and you will find it a delightful thing.

After a few hours' practice, it will come and stay for about ten
minutes. Then if you have practiced it and practiced it, it will come
and stay on a moment's notice. When I lecture here, I wait for this
state to come, because the words are not mine then. At that time,
you are in touch with the universe. You will ask no more
questions then of human beings.

All this will sound like a story until you have practiced and
practiced. You have a little glimpse of what it is. You have to stay
in it. This is the way you bring it first—by rhythmic breathing.

It has been called Prana. Those who called it Prana did not
experience it. This is in the body but it is not Prana. It is this
nectar, this Amiya. It is very thin, self-sufficient. It has no
awareness. When you are it, when you have become that, you have
no desire to find out what it is either. You are in it. It will keep you
eternally young. You cannot age because it is beyond time and
space. Time cannot enter into it. It is so powerful.

What man understands as power is dissipation of power.
Kinetic energy is just the dissipation of energy, the difference
between voltage and amperage.

Here is the source of the voltage. The deeper you go into the
voltage, it becomes so great you can't see it. (Like lightning.) The
deeper you go into it, if you wish something, it is more powerful
than the lightning and you can't help get the wish. On that
moment you can't be selfish because self does not exist. Everything has vanished. It is such a beautiful state. This is what we mean
by Amiya. It sounds very complex, but it is very simple the
moment you have experienced it.

If you experienced it once and can't get it back, it is because you experienced it accidentally. Now, do it consciously and you will find out how to bring it at will.

III.

SECRET OF YOUTH

You hear all sorts of advices about posture, how to learn to walk straight and how to carry yourself erect. You take all kinds of exercises to achieve this result, and if you do succeed in walking erect, you do so in a strained manner.

Now, there is one little secret of physiology that will give you correct posture in an instant. It is based on the research findings of our Institute.

We will not use any technical or Latin words to explain the physiology of what we are going to show you, but we shall ask you to experiment and find out the truth.

1.

Walk as you usually do across the room. You will notice you are bringing your entire weight down on your legs and feet. The noise of your steps will show this, as well as your feeling of *weight* as you walk.

2.

Next, we shall ask you to walk lightly. You will walk across the room as though you are walking on eggs, trying not to make any noise. That is walking carefully, but we have asked you to walk lightly.

How?

3.

Stand erect and try to lift yourself from the waist up, as though you are going to spring as a tiger or a cat. (The leap of the cheetah.)

Here you feel that the energy is coming from the *waist* and intercostal muscles going upward away from gravity. This sensation of lightness and sprightness is the key to rejuvenation.

4.

Now stand on your left foot and begin to swing your right limb from the hip. Feel the movement from the hip socket, not from the feet or limbs. Then stand on your right foot and swing your left limb from the hip in the same manner.

In this way you will learn you have a hip socket.

5.

You will now walk across the room by using your hip socket to propel your movement.

That is, do not walk with your whole weight on your feet and legs, but *walk lightly from the hips.*

Exaggerate the movement at first until you have learned the trick of walking from your hips.

You will notice when you walk from the hips that—

(1) Your abdomen *automatically* caves in, your chest *automatically* goes out, and your shoulders *automatically* become straight.

(2) You are making no sound with your feet.

(3) You have no sense of weight.

With no sense of effort or strained look of standing at attention, you are holding yourself erect and walking lightly without effort.

It is so easy. But you will slump back into your old habit the next moment. So you must practice, practice, practice, until it becomes your new habit.

Sit the same way, not slumped in your chair, but with a slight pull from the buttocks, as though you are about to get up.

Therefore, never sit down glued to earth, and never walk on earth to stay there slave of gravity, but simply alight on the ground, ready to take off at any moment. As you walk, get a feeling of flying—*scaling the air like a bird.*

The secret of rejuvenation in one word is the spring of life. Notice I am using the word *spring* in every sense of the word. Therefore, try to feel that spring.

This spring, physically speaking, comes from the pelvic up. Youth is from the waist up and old age is from the waist down. Carry yourself in walking, working, climbing, sitting down, all the time in the upper part of the body, lightly, like a feather, without holding the breath. In other words, don't try to practice this lightness by fighting and constriction, but laughingly, joyfully, and playfully feel the muscles, the neck and the head of the upper part of the body, light as vapor, and go on toward the objective. Here is the key to youth.

One more thing, as you walk, as you work, as you go about your daily tasks, keep your lower jaw relaxed and thus breathe easily, lightly, without effort, and smile—not a salesman's smile or grin, but the inward hormonic smile of *Amiya* (as explained in "Breath is Life").

IV.

WHAT IS ASTHMA?

Apart from the pathology, due to bacteria, we find that the asthma patient is lazy in his phrenic nerve, intercostal nerves, intercostal muscles, and diaphragm. The lymph nodes do not empty themselves and replace themselves normally enough. In one word, the diaphragm is a very lazy diaphragm.

First of all, we must know, what is asthma:

1. Asthma is a disease of breathing out.

2. Breathing out means preponderance of carbon dioxide.

3. The asthma patient pushes the carbon dioxide with tremendous force, through anxiety due to discomfort.

4. The asthma patient has a windpipe full of islands due to streptococci infection; many times a diphtheroid condition. As a rule, the vast populace of the United States is afflicted by staphylococci or streptococci infections due to kissing.

5. Thrombines coming through the blood vessels become entangled as the blood plates pass the rough spots. Continual clogging of the vascular system takes place. Therefore, with the least irritation by carbon dioxide, the nerves cause the vaso-constriction. Air, especially carbon dioxide, passing through this constricted area, causes asthma.

6. Smoking with its nineteen different kinds of poison, especially carbon monoxide, kills the tissue cells.

7. Continual cold infections aggravate the condition.

8. Asthma, let it be understood, is a diseased tissue condition. The carbon dioxide onrush aggravates this condition, causing clamping or vaso-constriction.

The remedy therefore is to stop irritating the diseased tissue by gushing carbon dioxide. No one wants to understand what I mean by gushing carbon dioxide. They do not want to understand because then they would have to change their life habits. They would much rather suffer through asthma, taking drug after drug, keep on propagandizing, and make life miserable.

Therefore, the remedy means very little to the asthma patient, because he will not change his habit of breathing out. If you have a sore spot in your body, you do not scratch it, but if you have a sore spot in your throat, you will scratch it with carbon dioxide, and that is called asthma.

Treatment: If you have an acute case of asthma, go at once to your doctor. He will give you a sedative to bring immediate relief. There are any number of drugs which will give immediate and temporary relief.

But if the doctor is not immediately available, what shall you do?

Open your mouth wide and hang out your tongue, even if you have to put your fist in your mouth to keep it open. *Take short, light breaths now through the mouth* (always with the mouth wide open) to relieve instantly.

All day long practice this, this sagging of the jaw and gentle breathing.

Now about the diseased tissue. Cure of any diseased tissue is fresh tissue begotten by cell division. Cell division takes place by circulation which will give fresh food to the cells to carry out the end-products. Therefore, we have got to reestablish gentle, sweet circulation in this diseased throat area locally.

The greatest enemy of circulation is emotion. Therefore, you have to become a smooth mental creature. To do this, you will sit in a fresh aired room and *smile through your whole being* and settle down in your mind, so that unconsciously your breathing becomes low, sweet and soft. This is not a salesman's smile but the thalmus smile described in "This Precious Heart."

As we said before, the asthma patient has a lazy diaphragm. Here the belly muscles have lost their normal muscle tone, because of fear that the exhalation might hurt the diseased tissue of the throat. Therefore a systemic treatment of a few months is absolutely necessary for regeneration.

Coffee, cigarettes, or any other excitant of the diseased condition of the throat tissue, must be eliminated. So also alcohol, and any irritant food, even too much salt, which will irritate the tissue, must be guarded against.

Above all, the diaphragm and the trachea are the local parts that must be oxidized by gentle exercises, which will twist the torso and work on the diaphragm and the intercostal muscles.

If your osteopath or doctor cannot give you exercises for regeneration, you must make up your mind to do it yourself, not by strenuous gymnastic exercises, which will only hurt these diseased tissues more, but by gentle, happy exercises involving the whole central nervous system, such as the scientific bioplays of life given in "Breath Is Life," "This Precious Heart" and the Extension Courses of our research institute.

Here a correlation takes place between the ancient sciences of the East and the modern sciences of the West in this new form of exercise known as the Acharyan bioplays of life designed to activate the cells of your entire body.

"Here life shall be being, living, but no longer breathing and unbreathing life, fighting resistance, and falling down in fatigue. Here life shall be a fight in peace.

Life shall be a smile forever."

A Strange Language

BREATH IS LIFE

INTRODUCTION TO PART FOUR

While the following account is not in any way meant to be a physiological treatise, its language is so vivid and dramatic that the physiology involved becomes very much alive. The idea behind the physiology is to show what we actually have to do to gain benefit from our breathing. The point that seems most important to me is that of rhythm and the mental attitude. Almost anything we do rhythmically with enjoyment seems to produce physical benefit.

The Pundit from his experience of Eastern philosophy and methods is in a good position to contribute to the phases where Western knowledge seems weakest. Taking breathing exercises without labor and trouble, but rather with the thought of inhaling honey from the air with the blessings of God in it, as expressed in the section called "Amiya in Oxygen," is typical of the Pundit Acharya's approach in his lectures and writings. Here we see physiology become sheer poetry.

In a previous work called *A Strange Language,* the Pundit Acharya took the very novel point of view that our body cells have a memory of their own and they also secrete a peculiar nectar or venom-hormone. What distinguishes the Pundit Acharya's work above all is his devotional attitude and his point of view that the *"Human Mind Is In Search Of Mind Of Matter."*

Wm. Harold Miller, M.D.

A WORD

While others blow the bugle of triumph reaping gold and glory from the kingdom of this their new Babylon,

And while they, in their ecstasy of victory, set fire to the earth and sky blinding the very vision of man—

Let me go on with my head bent low in all humility to my Master, sowing the seeds of beauty and life and hope on both sides of the Path,

For hath it not been said: "Thy Will be done on earth as it is in heaven."

I.

WHY WE BREATHE

Breath of Life

Through these pages we are passing on to you Meaningful Breathing.

The average person knows that breath is life. What he does not know is what is in the air that gives him life; and if he should find out what it is, his question would still be: how could he consciously use it?

A great many books and articles have been written about breathing. Also, in the name of Yoga many breathing exercises have been taught and practiced without any attention to the physiology of breathing.

Here, however, we record some conclusions based on the findings of our Institute. Some day we hope even the grammar schools of the world will teach the essence of these findings to the children and thus usher in a better human race.

Cells Are Live Animals

Now we learn to breathe anew! The moment we realize that it is not we who use the oxygen in the breath, but that every cell of the body does, we shall breathe differently.

First of all, the world of man must discover a new and very significant truth.

It is Mind of Matter. Not mind over matter. But Mind *of* Matter. It shall be man's revelation.

Cells are of matter. The chemistry of cells is elemental matter. The cells are all alive. Every one of the countless, uncounted number of different types of cells needs food. And oxygen is their chief food. It is *they* who breathe–The Cells!

Our effort in pulling in the air through the nose and sometimes through the mouth is effected by the cell-effort of the whole body. Ordinarily we are too lazy to help them do this. As a rule we let some of them have their oxygen but neglect the most of them.

In this new breathing man must remember these things:

1. It is the cells who have to get the oxygen from the breath.

2. If the cells do not work, they are not hungry.

3. If the cells do not eat and throw away their refuse (the end-product such as carbon dioxide), they die.

4. When cells die, we die because we are made up of cells.

5. Cells are tiny, so we must give them tiny beads of oxygen.

6. So our breathing effort must be very gentle and slow.

7. We must stir up every one of the cells in the body as we breathe in and out.

Basic Facts About Breathing

We are in charge of a zoo.

Our body and mind, meaning the brains, are composed of different types of tiny cells. They are different as to their structure and function, or work. Chiefly speaking, we have bone cells, muscle cells, tissue cells, gland cells, nerve cells, blood cells, and brain cells.

These cells eat by ingestion or absorption. All of them sleep or rest a part of each and every second, except the highest brain cells which are like batteries and become recharged only during a few hours of sleep. Up to a certain age of the individual the body-cells reproduce by cell division, after which only some of the cells, such as tissue cells, can increase in number. The brain cells never increase in number.

The most of the red cells of the blood die and are reborn every day.

We will not make this story of cells very complex. All we must remember is they have to have their food of protein, carbohydrate, fatty acids, oxygen, etc., so that they live, repair, produce heat, and cause activity of the body and mind. But the greatest of all food which they need all the time is *oxygen*.

The air we breathe is composed of approximately 77 percent nitrogen and 23 percent oxygen.

We breathe through the nose and mouth and it goes into the sacs called the lungs. In these sacs there are innumerable hairlike little tubes called capillaries. In these tender and soft capillaries, red cells of the blood separate the oxygen from the air by a chemical process. Here goes on the great laboratory work of nature.

Blood and Air

The blood goes through the entire body, including the brain cells, and supplies food and oxygen to the cells and takes the left-over carbon dioxide and brings it back to the lungs to be thrown out.

The red corpuscles in the blood give the oxygen to the cells. As soon as the carbon element of the cells has an exchange with the oxygen, the result is carbon dioxide, which is poisonous and which we breathe out.

Every minute the blood in the body passes through the hairlike capillaries of the lungs.

For just a second or two, the blood loses the carbon dioxide or poison, and some moisture. It gains the oxygen. The oxygen mixes with the crimson hemoglobin of the red cells in the blood. The hemoglobin becomes oxo-hemoglobin of scarlet color. At this moment of exchange the temperature is a little reduced.

Capacity of the Lungs

About two pints of air at the most can stay in the lungs all the time, which even by the greatest forced exhalation, cannot be thrown out.

An individual can take in and out a pint of air at every breath.

In the greatest forced breathing, one can suck in about two more pints, making three pints in all.

Therefore, it is five pints of air that one can play with.

But please bear in mind that one should not try any stunt breathing. Stunt breathing is done by expert Hatha-Yogis who experiment in the realm of physiology without any definite knowledge of biochemistry. Therefore ordinary people will only hurt themselves through vaso-constriction and tension caused by stunt breathing.

Ease and *Enjoyment* of the fresh air should be the keynotes of gentle and deep breathing.

II.

HOW WE BREATHE

Delicate Mechanism of Feeding

We are trying to make a very simple story out of the very complex mechanism of circulation and oxidation. With a little patience the average person will understand this story better if he will study this book over and over again.

The blood flows through vessels or tubes, each set being successively finer in structure. These are known as arteries, veins, venules, arterioles, and capillaries. Therefore the blood cannot come in direct contact with the cells. What does happen is, through the sides of these tubes through which the blood flows, food materials and oxygen ooze out to a little salty liquid like colorless water bathing the cells.

This fluid is lymph. This fluid passes through the body along with the blood by the side of miles of blood vessels, etc. It is the lymph fluid that gives food and oxygen to the cells. Instantly the lymph takes out the carbon dioxide or other refuse from the cells and puts it back into the blood stream. The blood brings back carbon dioxide, the poisonous material, to the lungs to be thrown out. This makes the picture very simple to us.

So we shall remember that the body is continually playing with the lymph fluid. Pressure on the abdominal muscles, etc., is pushing the lymph fluid to the chest cavity, where there are many ducts (canals) to which they must come to get their fresh supply of oxygen. As we breathe out, the chest cavity presses the lymph fluid down to other parts of the body.

In breathing in and out, we shall only remember then, the

pushing in and out of lymph fluids to and from the chest cavity.

Thus, as we breathe in, the lymph fluid is coming to the chest cavity, and as we are breathing out, the lymph fluid is going along with the blood to various parts of the body to feed the cell animals.

In breathing therefore, when we suggest the particular exercises of breathing, we must remember that we are trying to bring the lymph fluid to the chest cavity in inhalation (breathing in), and pushing the lymph fluid out of the chest cavity to other parts of the body in exhalation (breathing out). There are ducts in the thoracic or chest cavity where the lymph is sucked in during inhalation and is pushed away in exhalation. We shall call upon our memory and refer to this mechanism while taking our practical exercises.

The thing to remember here shall be, it is the lymph fluid that gives the plasma to the living cells. Secondly, the lymph fluid is continually passing things in and out of the blood vessels. Thirdly, blood and lymph are present everywhere in the body. And lastly, life is the *Stirring up of Lymph Fluid* that it may run in a smooth flow.

Therefore, gentle stirring.

It is true that lymph is bathing the living cells, and blood is in capillaries present everywhere in the body. Therefore, it is actually the pushing of the blood to the chest cavity rather than the lymph, which is the process of inspiration. But the entire physiological process will be too complex for the layman, so we shall only speak of working with the lymph fluid.

The Laws of Oxidation

The taking of this food and giving up of carbon dioxide by the cells is oxidation. Let us have a picture of the burning of fuel and throwing out of ashes. Only ashes in this case is the gas known as carbon dioxide.

If we do not work, we are not hungry. The cells are likewise not hungry if they do not work. And the more they work, the more food they need. This process is simple to understand.

Every time the cells work, oxidation takes place. The result is action and heat. Every time the cells work, the potential energy sleeping within the cells becomes expressed energy (kinetic). The result is, the energy is dissipated: one-third in action and two-thirds in heat. Thus the body gets its heat. This radiation is dissipated as the skin gives off the heat.

In the process of this cell oxidation, electrical sparks are generated. Thus currents of electricity are going through the body.

This electricity is life. The end-product or leftover of this oxidation is this gas, carbon dioxide.

What Causes Breathing

In the neck of the individual there is a reflex spot called the respiratory center. From this center there runs a set of nerves which excites the lungs.

Now, as the scarlet blood rich in oxygen and just leaving the oxygen-filled lungs is going through the great big thick arteries of the body, the red corpuscles in it are giving food and oxygen to the cells and gathering carbon dioxide, the garbage. Then the blood passes through the big veins. This venous blood has become purple with carbon dioxide, the end-product.

When this carbon dioxide becomes too much, it causes acidity in the blood. This acidity releases the hydrogen ion in the blood, and this hydrogen when it touches the respiratory center in the neck excites the nerves running from there to the thoracic cavity and diaphragm. There you have the beginning of the enlarging of the thoracic (or chest) cavity, and the inflated chest cavity immediately causes pulling in of the air through the nose, breathing in.

Now, from the walls of the lungs to the center in the neck, there runs another contradictory set of nerves called vagii, which causes deflation of the chest cavity, and thereby we breathe out.

Panting

Now we can understand that when we are running, more

carbon dioxide is generated in the body and more hydrogen is released, causing increased activity of the chest cavity in quick succession. Thus, the individual pants.

In other words, when one is working hard or running, the cells of the body are eating up oxygen quickly. Also they are throwing out more carbon dioxide in quick succession. And more carbon dioxide is releasing the hydrogen, and the hydrogen is going to the neck and exciting the nerves that inflate the chest cavity. So we have a quick up and down movement of the chest cavity like a bellows.

Now stop running and you have stopped quick oxidation or eating and throwing off of garbage by the cells. So panting has come back to normal or slower breathing.

Breathing Mechanism

We know, if we run an automobile in jerks, by giving a jerky gas supply to the carburetor, the motor does not last long. Similarly, when we have jerky action among the cells by jerky breathing in and out, we have abnormal conditions in the body.

One does not need very much imagination to see what is happening in the body.

A little while ago we talked about the spot in the neck. In the neck there is the portion of the anatomy through which all the nerves of the brain are running to the body through a place called the medulla oblongata.

In this medulla oblongata in the neck is a center called the vital knot. From this knot are going two sets of nerves to all parts of the body, whose branches fall on the walls of the blood vessels of the internal organs, such as the heart, lungs, stomach, intestines, colon, etc.

One set of these nerves is called vaso-constrictor nerves, that is, those which cause constriction or contraction of the blood vessels, etc. Another set of nerves is called vaso-dilator nerves, which cause dilation or enlargement of the blood vessels.

The moment one holds one's breath, there is more carbon dioxide or poison held in the body. And that moment there is constriction in different organic parts of the body due to the excitement of these vaso-constrictor nerves by the carbon dioxide poison.

These nerves therefore are like the brakes of an automobile. One cannot run an engine of a car by fooling with the brakes and giving spasmodic gas. If one does, one will not have a car very long.

Common sense tells a driver how to drive his car smoothly by giving a regular flow of gas instead of jerky gas, and putting the brakes on and off gently instead of in jerky motions. But the average human being has not enough common sense to do that much for his own body and brain.

What is said in these few lines is so very important that it concerns the very life and death of human beings.

Even highly developed intellectual human beings may not have enough horse sense to drive the machine of their bodies and minds smoothly with the flow of carbon dioxide and blood and lymph fluid. In this work our aim is to teach man that much about his body which he must know in order to live healthily and happily.

Rhythmic Breathing

We have different planes of action and consciousness.

Let us see. When a person is resting quietly, his breathing is low. Then when he is thinking and still resting, his vague emotional moods are quickening his breaths. This is the normal plane of life and thoughts.

Now, as he gets up and begins to work physically, along with his thoughts his breath quickens still more. This is the second plane of action and thought.

Then we take an extreme case where a person is running or hurrying rapidly through some work with tremendous excitement of his body and thoughts. His breaths become very rapid and short. This is the third or extreme plane of action and thought. It is like an automobile going ninety miles an hour.

Now, one can go at a tremendous speed and yet not hurt himself if the breathing is rhythmic, because in all rhythmic breaths the flow of blood and lymph is always normal, meaning never obstructed by vaso-constriction and tension. If one learns to run in such a way that he will not cause any vaso-constriction, the flow of life will go on smoothly.

There is no end to the follies of human breathing. Perfect breathing, whether slow or rapid, should be regular, meaning the first breath should equal the second, the second one the third, and so on. Perfectly, in terms of fractions of seconds.

Perfect breathing has never been seen even in sleep. Five minutes of regular rhythmic breathing, even in sleeping people, is a rare vision.

Only in Samadhi the Yogi has perfect breathing. Because life at last is in contact with the fount of life.

III.

BREATHING EXERCISES

We shall further explain this breathing mechanism at the end of the story. In the meanwhile we give you some definite exercises which will benefit you every day.

Proper breathing, when it becomes a new habit, will regenerate the cells of the tissues. It will teach you how to relax properly. It will make you sleep well. It will rejuvenate the whole body and mind by stirring up and rearranging all the necessary "ions" of the body. Proper breathing will help you in digestion and elimination. After a few months of proper breathing, you will find results which will make you grateful to this little book.

Here are three definite exercises which we suggest to every man, woman and child.

Exercise i

1.

Stand or sit or lie down straight, so that the spinal cord and the head are in a straight line.

2.

With infinite slowness and gentleness, and mind you, it has got to be with infinite slowness and gentleness, start to take a deep breath.

The moment we say, deep breath, we know you will start to hurry. This hurry will cause vaso-motor constriction. This will spoil the whole thing. It will hurt you. It is better not to take the breathing exercises at all, than to take a breath with constriction.

Therefore, again we say, with infinite gentleness and slowness– a thing that modern human beings do not know.

Again we say, *with infinite gentleness and slowness*—because this is the key to the whole situation—start to take a slow, deep breath. Imagine as though you are holding a tray of ashes before your nose. You must breathe in and out so gently but deeply as not to cause the ashes to be disturbed.

3.
Now, contract the muscular walls of the abdomen, lift the ribs, and expand the chest cavity as you breathe in.

4.
Mentally draw a circle around your waist underneath the navel. From there, feel as though you are pulling a tree up, root and all. Likewise pull the abdominal cavity in, and pull the whole body from the waist up, as you take in this breath, enlarging the chest cavity all around.

Beware! Do it slowly and gently. Remember the ashes on the tray.

5.
In breathing, lift up the shoulders and send the air to the upper part of the lungs (apex) which, through neglect and laziness, becomes the seat of tuberculosis and pneumonia.

6.
While you are taking the breath, look out that your neck and face and eyes do not get tight.

7.
Therefore, while you are breathing in, that is, during the entire breathing-in period, keep on smiling, so that the head and neck and face and eyes will remain completely relaxed.

8.
This is the Secret of Breathing: No constriction is allowed in breathing in.

9.

After you have taken in a breath, exhale or send it out just as slowly and gently.

As you walk through the streets all day long, practice this every so often so that you form the habit, and until this habit becomes your second nature.

Your objective should be to make your waist slender like that of a tiger. If you are fat, this will start to reduce you by increasing the metabolism of your body. If you are slender, this will make you strong.

After fifty or sixty of such breaths, you will feel completely relaxed. Gradually and gradually your whole body chemistry will revitalize itself, bringing about freshness and rejuvenation.

Exercise ii

Early in the morning, before you rise out of bed, please create this new habit.

1.

If you have to get up at eight o'clock in the morning, wake up at seven o'clock.

2.

Open your eyes and lie quiet in bed. Never get up in a hurry.

3.

Slowly, very slowly, with infinite slowness, start to yawn.

4.

Slowly turn and twist your body with infinite slowness and gentleness. Wring and twist the body like you would wring a towel.

5.

Stretch your arms and legs, and turn and twist your body from the pelvis to the neck, while keeping relaxed in the neck and head.

6.

With every turn and twist, take a soft deep breath. Inhale and exhale, and turn and twist, and stretch and turn. Make the body as supple as that of a reptile.

7.

Take one inch of muscle at a time mentally, and stretch it and pull it away from the ribs and the bones. Feel as though the flesh is being pulled out from the bones. You must feel it.

8.

Warning: If you do too much horse-riding the first day, you will have sore muscles and backache. Similarly, if you do too much of this the first day, you will have sore muscles and backache too.

If you are not patient and slow with these exercises, you will have sad results. Therefore, we advise you to do this a little at a time, until your body is completely broken and has become supple.

The aim is to stir up the lymph fluid and oxidation in every part of the body, a little at a time, stirring up and revitalizing all the ions of the body. The aim is to awaken the vitality of every cell of the body, neglecting not even one.

The one thing that you must remember while so doing is that the nerve cells of the neck and the brain cells must be kept calm and cool.

Therefore, in these exercises one must learn how to enjoy this feeling of the body through and through. Every time you turn and twist and yawn, and take a breath and breathe out, enjoy the honey in the body. Turn the sensual enjoyment into a sensuous delicacy.

Begin to feel the glory of youth and exhilaration of life itself. With this soft prayer on your lips in the morning:

"Love, I am glad to be alive in the same world with you."

Exercise iii

In winter many people have cold feet and take hot water bottles to bed. People also have cold hands and face. There are people whose vitality is very low due to low metabolism. All these people should learn how to take this exercise of breathing through the feet and hands and the whole body.

The plants breathe through the green of their leaves. The fishes breathe through their gills. Potatoes and onions breathe through their skin by ingesting oxygen or carbon dioxide, as their need be.

The cells of the human body are tiny animals. They too breathe whether man breathes or not. Many people have to put their hands out in bed or their hands suffocate. We do not cover the entire face and keep only the nose open to breathe at night, because the cells of the face breathe independently of the nose. It is all a question of habit.

Today man must learn again how to breathe through his hands and feet. The process is simple:

1.

Pull in air through the feet first, the same as you do through the nose, while breathing through the nose. Put your attention on the feet and feel the pull of air through the bottom of the feet.

2.

Pull the air in through the legs and the whole body. Gradually you will find that your feet are getting warmer, oxidation and radiation taking place. What is happening is that you are stirring up the lymph fluid in those muscles and the skin, and the cell muscles are getting their food. In other words, it is the local work that is needed.

The cell animals are alive. They have a life of their own. You are teaching them again to do their own work independently of the body. You are beginning to live by inches of your body. Your body is becoming alive by inches.

3.

Now do the same thing with your hands. Learn to breathe through them. That is, pull the air through the palm of your hand the same as you do through your nose.

4.

Send the air through the whole arm and body rhythmically, as you are doing through the nose.

5.

Now breathe through the whole body. Let all the cells of your body be vibrant with oxidation.

6.

Early in the morning when you get up, stand erect on the floor in bare feet and do this exercise, and you will be a new creature for the rest of the day.

7.

During the day when you are very active, take a couple of minutes off from your work and do this exercise every so often, and you will feel refreshed.

In the physical exercises that you do and in the physical work that you perform, you do not let the entire body have the flow of this oxidation. You exercise your body in jerks. The result is, there are creases left in the body where no oxygen can enter. This is the part of the body which becomes subject to germ diseases and atrophication. These are the parts of the body which will kill you.

Therefore, keep no creases in the body. Let the plumbing of your nerves and circulatory system, these arteries, veins, and nerves, enjoy the rhythmic flow of life in work or rest.

You will begin to be a new creature.

Dangerous Breathing Exercises

You have probably read or heard of many Hatha-Yoga stunts and exercises of dog-breathing, cat-breathing, or breathing while standing on the head, and so on. In this respect, you have only to remember that:

The tiny capillaries which take the oxygen from the lungs are so tiny and so thin and so delicate that they look just like human hair.

If you keep that in mind, and also that the cells of the body which take the oxygen and use it up are tiny little animal lives, you will understand why breathing exercises should be very gentle, while the entire body enjoys the flow and relaxation.

Never believe in any stunts of the body while breathing. There should be no constriction inside or outside of the body, and the blood and lymph fluid must flow very gently without causing any high blood pressure.

Any breathing exercise that will excite the head is dangerous. Any exercise that will bring constriction in the nerves is dangerous. Any exercise that will cause tightness in the neck is fatal to the life of the tiny animal cells, and therefore to the life and well being of your whole body.

Whatever the contortionist of the body does is not very healthy for the average human body or brain. You will not find a contortionist very healthy or happy in life. An acrobat of breathing exercises might be capable of doing some great stunts that we admire, but certainly it will not prevent him from being a victim of pneumonia, pleurisy or other diseases. It does not help his digestive or alimentary processes. Standing on the head, or breathing in dog posture, or violent ejection of breath by forced exhalation, will show the nerves of the face swollen.

Avoid all such exercises as you would poison.

Remember, life should be a continual rhythmic flow. As the ebb and tide of the ocean. As the entire solar universe and universes go on in rhythmic motion.

Jerks of action or thought are destructive to man.

Flow of blood and lymph and breath and thought are life and inspiration.

Breath is Life

In saying that breath is life, we are not becoming poetic.

To find out just exactly what we mean, experiment with breath and you will find out the meaning of the breath.

Exercise i

Suppose you have a cold. You have taken a physic. You have further taken some alkaline fruit juices or mild medicine. Still you are feeling not up to the mark.

Now, sit by an open window where a current of fresh air is flowing freely. Slowly and gently lift your head, straighten up, sit erect, and begin to take regular and rhythmic, deep, gentle breaths for half an hour. Smile and relax completely as you are breathing.

You will find, hot or cold weather outside, that you are beginning to feel warmer and warmer, until you begin to sweat.

Stop for an hour or so. Then take another half hour's similar exercise.

Wait an hour or two. Once more take the same exercise for another half hour, and you will find your cold is beginning to disappear.

Exercise ii

Suppose you get up with an acid condition in your body. You are feeling sluggish. It is probably gloomy or rainy outside. You have no ambition. Everything is going around in your head. You feel heavy and stuffy.

Again sit for an hour at a time before the open window and take these exercises.

You will find in a short while you are rejuvenated. All heaviness is gone and you feel light as air. The world is beautiful again and you are ready to do your work.

Therefore, breath is a new inspiration.

Exercise iii

Suppose your digestive process is out of order. You do not feel hungry, or if you eat, you suffer from gas.

Take these exercises:

Sit before an open window or in the open air, and stir up all the abdominal region during your breathing.

Do it once, twice, thrice during the day, or in bed before you go to sleep, and you will find a tremendous change occurring in your metabolic processes.

What, then, does breath do?

To understand it, one must understand the philosophy of the human body.

The human body with its various organs and nerves, contains all the elements that are in Nature, all the chemicals that could possibly be in a drug or pure food store. Scientifically speaking, all that can be found in the universe is in the human body. The cells arrange and rearrange, the blood arranges and rearranges, and the cell secretions arrange and rearrange all the elements, ions in the body, to bring about the very process of life.

It is laziness of the body and mind, therefore, which fails to take proper, regular breathing which causes the inertia and the acidity of the body. If this laziness and inertia keep up, the body gradually degenerates and atrophy sets in in different parts of the body.

Breathe deeply and gently through every cell of the body, laugh happily, and release the head of all worries and anxieties; and finally, breathe in the blessing of love, hope, and immortality that is flowing in the air, and you will understand the meaning of human breath.

Life is in the air and air is in the body.

Breath therefore is divine breath.

To know it one must taste it.

To know the thing you have to be the thing.

Lazy Oxygen

We have told throughout the entire book that you must relax completely and smile while taking all these breathing exercises, for this scientific reason:

The cells of the body take the oxygen. That is, the carbon element in the cell body comes in contact with the oxygen element of the air. But the carbon cannot take the oxygen unless something happens to the cell itself.

The nitrogen element in the cell body, which is like nitrogen in nitro-glycerine in a bomb, must explode first so that a spark of fire will burn up the carbon and oxygen together, so that the oxidation may take place. This is what we have called "eating" by the cells.

In the cell body there are little bits of radio-gens which are like match sticks, causing the first spark of fire, thus enabling the carbon to be inflamed to burn the oxygen into an active oxygen atom.

This spark of radio-gen, causing the bursting out of the nitrogen of the cell, from the psychological standpoint, is called Will.

Now, when a person smiles and is relaxed, the Will functions better, so that the radio-gens can readily cause the bursting out of the cell body.

The subject matter sounds so complex that, if one wants to study it in a simple way, one would do well to read the most illuminating book on the subject: *Phenomenon of Life* by Dr. George Crile.

In breathing through the whole body, one has to stir up every cell of the body so that every cell of the body turns the lazy oxygen into active oxygen. Therefore, there should be present the birth of Will on the part of the cells themselves.

This Will of the cells in biology is called cell effort. It is the effort of the cells which brings about the sparks of electrons which cause the cells to be hungry for the oxygen.

Therefore one has to relax his brain, stop thinking and examining what is happening in the body, and let the cells of the body do the work. It calls for cell autonomy and cell volition. It presupposes that every living cell of the body should be told by the mind to do its own work while the mind looks on with a smile.

Should the mind be anxious to take in more oxygen through the air and use it up by swift or jerky activity of the body, involving the lungs and the heart, there would be constriction from the neck which would hamper the very work that the mind wants to do effectively. It is important therefore that the mind take a vacation and allow the body to breathe. The more the mind will interfere with the body, the less the body will breathe.

Emotional Breaths

There is one type of breathing that kills human beings more than anything else. That is the choking and interrupted breathing during emotions.

Hate, anger, fear, anxiety, depression, grief, and all other negative emotions cause choking and interrupted breathing. Sometimes they cause high blood pressure and alternately low blood pressure. Sometimes they hold the carbon dioxide too long in the body, thereby causing an acid condition, and often the body is too tired to take in the necessary oxygen. Either way it kills the person.

Therefore, the student must have a yardstick by which he may always judge whether his body is normal and healthy or not.

Two Yardsticks of Breathing

Catch yourself at any given moment and see if your head is hot or not. If it is, smile and drop the load of thoughts and anxiety from your head with a smile.

Yes, just break in a smile until the head has become cool.

While your head is hot, you will notice your breath is interrupted. You will also notice, as you are dropping the load from your head and neck, your breath has become normal again.

These are the two yardsticks which will enable you to bring health and happiness in your life. You will live to be a real person.

We do not care what is your life, what is your faith, that is, what is your occupational consciousness or your attitude toward other fellows and God.

One law you must obey. Flow along with cool breath and you will live. Stumble along with jerky breath and you die.

Smile and you live. Drop the smile and you die.

IV.

DIVINE BREATH

Why Smile

We have previously suggested that one should take a breath, meaning inhale and exhale, with the least amount of excitement. That is, one should do it very slowly and gently.

The scientific reason for this is:

1. The blood is running through the entire body, no part being neglected. It goes through thick arteries, then veins and other small blood vessels.

2. By a law of pressure and diffusion the food material and oxygen are leaking out from the blood vessels to the lymph fluid, and the lymph fluid is giving the food and oxygen to the cells. From the cells the lymph fluid is taking the carbon dioxide and other refuse and putting this garbage back into the blood stream, by the same law of pressure and diffusion in chemistry. The pressure and diffusion are called Osmosis and Dialysis.

3. Now in the vital knot of the neck there is a center which is called the Vaso-Motor Center. From there to most of the walls of the blood vessels run the nerve fibers that make up the cell-walls of the blood vessels. These vaso-motor nerve fibers are of two types:

(1)   Vaso-Constrictor Nerves

(2)   Vaso-Dilator Nerves

4. With excitement in the Vaso-Motor Center, the Vaso-Constrictor nerve fibers of the walls of the blood vessels clamp up the vessels and cause constriction, and the blood flow is interrupted. *This causes high blood pressure.*

We can easily see how with the least excitement of thoughts, especially emotions, the Vaso-Motor Center is excited, because with emotional excitement there is more activity of the body. More activity of the body calls upon most of the cells to oxidize and radiate heat. Thereby, they are creating more carbon dioxide. The more carbon dioxide there is, the more the acidity of the blood which releases hydrogen ion, the hydrogen ion exciting the respiratory center which causes inflation of the chest or thoracic cavity. That means a quick succession of intakes of breath or choking. Emotional activities are creating and holding carbon dioxide in the body too long.

Therefore, if one could inhibit this Vaso-Motor Center in the medulla oblongata in the neck, one could bring release at this point definitely and locally, so that there would be general relaxation in the body.

Now you see the necessity of subjectively bringing about a sense of release in the head and neck by a gentle smile so that vaso-dilation may take place. If you enjoy the sense of breathing, while breathing, you will automatically feel like smiling.

The attention should be not to watch the breathing, but to enjoy it. Oxygen is life. So to be happy and healthy, one must enjoy it.

Breathing exercises, therefore, should be taught to laymen by an expert operator of this science with a thorough knowledge of physiology, biochemistry, and objective experience, or man will never know the meaning of the breath.

It is regrettable that in the name of Yoga a great deal of advice has been given to laymen which is more harmful than beneficial. Some day the departments of Physiology and Neurology in the reputable universities of the world may establish departments of objective knowledge where Yoga breathing will be properly taught.

One may easily see how a suggestion should be made to such

institutions to introduce a mechanism which, with all biochemical and physiological references involved, will enable the students to fully grasp the meaning of human breathing.

Breath, meaning oxygen, is so vital to life that in this civilized day and age this study is of primary importance to humanity and should not be left in the hands of "Coney Island Psychologists" in or outside of academic circles.

Disease of The Will

The greatest difficulty the individual finds in learning correct breathing is lack of the Will. The average normal person does not know to what extent he is subject to the slavery of his habits.

The body wants to act automatically while the mind wants to go astray in meaningless thoughts of the day. As a fad, one may take a few correct breaths for one day, and then forget all about it.

Therefore, there is the necessity of the Will to will.

It may sound harsh, but years of experience have brought us to the conclusion that one has to hold a mental whip over his mind to Will.

This is a very unpleasant and unpopular process. To Will effectively, one has to whip the will and keep on doing so. We know we are asking for the impossible, yet this alone can give one normal health and happiness.

The task is all the more difficult because even the educated people of the world pay so little attention to the practice of proper breathing.

But we are in a new age where Man's consciousness is finding itself and reaching for the stars.

Therefore, we know that the new man with this new consciousness will find this will and keep on willing it.

It is so easy to enjoy life without constriction. But poor man makes it so hard for himself by straining his central nervous system with habitual irregular breath.

This philosophy with practical applications, taught by members of an expert institute of objective knowledge, where love for man and not money or glory is the objective, shall be given even to children in the grammar schools so that we shall have a better human race.

Psychological reproach of man for his wild and chaotic thinking and ways of living is of no avail. He must learn the ways of biochemistry so that he will be able to control his own consciousness of the body and mind.

Strange Causes of Vaso-Constriction

We have suggested, somewhat vaguely, how the nerve fibers of the Vaso-Constrictor nerves running to the walls of the blood vessels cause Vaso-Constriction. We have also suggested how Constriction is responsible for the generation of too much carbon dioxide, causing acidity in the blood, and subsequent holding of the breath and choking.

In a later book we shall show how the interruption of the digestive process, and derangement and interruption of the alimentary process, as well as constipation, are effected by similar causes. But here we shall answer the possible inquiries of the student which might justly be raised as to the causes of this Vaso-Constriction.

The cause of Constriction by the excitation of the center in the neck is mental, that is, emotional.

It starts with the arousal of an instinct known as Pugnacity. Pugnacity gives rise to the emotion of anger. Constriction also is aroused by the instinct of flight with its subsequent emotion of fear.

There is a definite chemical secretion by the brain cells which brings about these instinctive and emotional responses.

The story is too deep and too intricate even for an ordinary book of Physiology or Neurology.

It remains, therefore, for us to reveal the findings of the Institute, based upon objective experience in the study of the mental processes of the average man and woman. These findings should contribute to the pages of a new science of Neuro-Electronics.

Here are some of the suggestions:

1.   We start with the so-called inanimate kingdom. We see a type of stone called Stinkstone. When this stone is decomposed into organic matter, it gives out a definite stink or bad odor.

2.   Stinkweed (as Jimson Weed, Ailanthus, etc.) and similar types of weeds do the same thing.

3.   Stinkwood functions likewise.

4.   Stinkhorn (of the order of Phallales, especially Ithyphallus imphudicus of ill-smelling fungi) functions in the same manner.

5.   Then we have various types of bugs of the order of Hemiptra which give out a bad odor in the process of their protection against the enemy.

6.   Cobras and many other snakes secrete and pour out a venom acid for protection in fear and hate.

7.   Mosquitoes do likewise.

8.   Scorpions have their stings.

9.   The Skunk generates a fearful acid and sprays it in fear and hate.

10.   The Bedbug gives out an obnoxious acid when one tries to hurt it.

In other words, starting with the color variations of the insects and birds, which are brought about by cell secretion in protection and adaptation to inevitability, and as we study the stink acid secretions of flora and fauna, we find that nature has a stinking or biting weapon to protect itself.

Human brain cells which are the last great, great, great, great grandchildren of these biological stones, weeds, woods, bugs, reptiles, etc., have inherited the skunk juice or the bedbug juic/ hormones. As soon as the basic instinct of pugnacity or flight aroused, they secrete the skunk or bedbug juice hormones.

The result is an immediate acidity of the blood.

Physiology has made a mistake in assuming that the Adrena Medullas with the small Adrenals of the spine, as well as thyroic secretions, alone cause all emotions. These glandular juices only inflame the cells to actuate and keep on actuating in the secretion of this poisonous hormone that we are suggesting. It is not glandular secretions that cause the moods and emotions, but a definite cell secretion of this type that is the beginning of the process of emotion.

In a separate volume, *A Strange Language*, in a chapter dealing with Amiya and Hala-Hal, we have suggested that the cell secretions change with every mood of the human brain. These secretions are not accidental but identical with the need of the whole organism.

Here we shall only suggest very mildly that every negative and destructive emotional mood and thought of man causes the brain cells' secretion of the skunk and bedbug juice hormone which immediately touches upon the Vaso-Motor Center in the neck with ensuing Constriction.

Whenever we see an argumentative person, either vocal or silent, we know that the brain cells of such a person are secreting this juice, and he or she is suffering from attacks of the instincts of Pugnacity and Flight. The only thing that will bring such a person back to a normal condition is neutralization or alkalization of this skunk secretion in the brain.

Oxygen alone can neutralize this juice.

Lazy oxygen cannot be digested by the cells unless there is a hunger on the part of these cells.

Smile alone will give the release to the cells which will restore their normal hunger for oxygen.

Smile therefore neutralizes the skunk or bedbug juice of the brain cells.

Whenever this venom secretion is in the brain, (and it is so common with the average person that he always starts a sentence with a "but"), he is holding his breath and suffering from carbon dioxide in so doing.

Smile and oxygen—oxygen and smile—are the immediate remedy, the alkalization of such a lost sheep.

God must send his Son anew to teach man how to smile and give up his "buts."

No book of Physiology or Neurology has gone into this subject which is of such vital importance to humanity. It is regrettable that the essential secrets of life are not taught to human beings by the learned men of the Science of Life. The average man is left in the hands of "quacks" who give him all types of panaceas but the right one.

This finding of the cell secretion of a type of skunk or bedbug juice is of supreme importance. It is not to be laughed at or taken lightly.

When man understands this he will be the beginning of the new psychic species. The Man of Tomorrow.

As soon as a creative impulse is present in matter, the cells of plants and animals and the brain cells secrete Amiya, the nectar. But as soon as the destructive impulses appear in it, Hala-Hal or venom, or skunk juice, is secreted by them.

More than that.

The food is being cooked. It gives a delicious, savory aroma. It is digestible.

The food burns. It gives out an awful odor. It is poisonous.

Somewhere there is a fire. Disintegration of matter. It stinks.

A streak of lightning goes through space rending the nitrogen atoms from the oxygen. The earth is going to get its nitrogen.

The space is filled with honeyed air.

Then again, spring and love that bring the hope of life smell sweet. Spring is creative.

Death smells. Ask the neighborhood dog. The cat leaves home when death is about to appear.

On the other hand, cooing pigeons dance around in joy when love like a rose blooms.

Perfume is identified with life itself. An awful odor is the sign of death.

Matter and mind secrete both venom and nectar—venom with the appearance of disintegration or death, and nectar when the god of life calls on youth and love and hope.

Immortality therefore is all nectar.

Smile Is Not a Grin

We have said that when you take in a breath, that is, during the entire period of your inhalation, you should smile, so that there will be no vaso-constriction. You think you know what we mean by smile.

No.

The human smile is motivated by a lurking anticipation of an immediate or remote reward, however hidden the impulse may be. No one smiles except for a social reason. The human smile is an exchange of give-and-take philosophy between man and man or man and woman.

We do not mean this smile. We do not mean the type of smile evidenced by the sign you see in business offices: Keep on smiling.

Our smile is a process of dropping the thoughts from the head. It is like the shedding of the leaves of a tree in autumn. It is like discarding a soiled garment after a bath. This smile is a shower-bath.

One should learn a smile which will redeem him and release him from the consciousness of all solid, liquid, gas, electricity, and all other forms of matter. It is like the sense of relief of a sigh which says: "Thank God, it's all over."

It is a sense of freedom. Complete freedom. Therefore, it is a pale happiness that is so pale that even a mist or fading smoke is too heavy in comparison. This smile has no more desire. This smile starts where desires end.

Amiya in Oxygen

We have promised to give you a revelation.

In the bosom of the oxygen atom there is a hidden essence not to be detected by human eye. This is its very soul. It is Amiya or nectar.

It is this nectar which combines with the essence of the carbon atom of the human cells that expresses itself in the form of the electrical sparks of life, which is human energy.

Do you want to find it?

Sit alone by a window before the sunrise in the morning, where a cool, gentle breeze is flowing before and around you.

Without stirring even a ray of thought in your brain, breathe softly. You will find an elixir of honeyed nectar in the perfumed air which you are breathing. Do not try to watch it, for it will degrade into solid matter again and the essence will be lost.

Do you want to find it more?

The blessings of the entire Nature and God are in this air that is free from mercury, dust, and all other impurities of the day. Beneath the infinite sky above, and the limitless space before you, in the soft twilight of the dawn, as the cool breeze kisses your brow, like the gentle caress of a mother's affectionate gaze, try to breathe gently, very gently, infinitely gently, this pale air, and you will find the Amiya of the gods in the oxygen.

It is this Amiya which is the essence of life.

It is ever present in the solar universe.

Lucky is the man who would understand it, and mutely, in grateful recognition bow his head to his Maker and say:

"Thank you, Love, for giving me this life every day, every hour, every minute of my existence."

Go out alone in the woodland in spring and you will see every leaf, every twig of the trees and plants and vines and shrubs, green in the joy of being, ever grateful to this Amiya for giving it life.

Sit by a brook or a stream, and in the songs of the brooks and rivers and lakes you will hear them sing the glory of life while ravishing waters dance with Amiya in water and air.

Go out in the purple dusk of the sunset and you will find the earth and the mountains and the seas and the sky–all bent in audible whispers of prayer that life goes on ever and ever with this omnipresent air.

Close your eyes and you will find in the heart of your heart the fount spring of this nectar which alone is life and all else is death.

Everywhere you look there is air.

There is light. There is sound. There is soft touch. Caress of love.

There is love in the air. Blessings of Buddha, Moses, Christ and all the souls who have blessed Man.

Breathe of this life, love, hope and blessings, and bend your head in gratitude.

For breath is life.

And love flows in and out with every breath.

Breath is but the Divine Breath.

THE WORKS OF BUBBA FREE JOHN

THE KNEE
OF LISTENING
The Early Life and Radical
$3.95   *Spiritual Teachings of Franklin Jones*

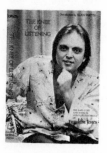

In September, 1970, after thirteen years of intense sadhana, Bubba Free John (Franklin Jones) permanently realized the condition of unqualified God-consciousness.

During the next year he wrote *THE KNEE OF LISTENING: The Early Life and Radical Spiritual Teachings of Franklin Jones*, which describes his spiritual odyssey and contains the basic statements of his radical dharma, the path of Understanding.

In April, 1972, The Dawn Horse Communion was established. The formal teaching of Bubba Free John had begun. During the first two years of the Ashram's existence, Bubba spoke frequently on many fundamental aspects of spiritual life, but he always returned to the subject of Satsang, the transforming relationship between Guru and disciple, which is the primary instrument of all true Spiritual Masters. The most powerful and instructive of these talks have been compiled in Bubba's second book, *THE METHOD OF THE SIDDHAS: Talks with Franklin Jones on the Spiritual Technique of the Saviors of Mankind.*

From March through July, 1974, Bubba generated in his Ashram a series of extraordinary events that forcefully illustrated both his Divine nature and the radical, all-inclusive nature of his dharma. The events of this period and the teaching relative to them have been chronicled in *GARBAGE AND THE GODDESS: The Last Miracles and Final Spiritual Instructions of Bubba Free John.*

With the completion of *Garbage and the Goddess*, Bubba announced that his primary teaching work in the world was done. He continues to speak and write, but the fundamental communication of the radical path of Understanding is contained in these three books.

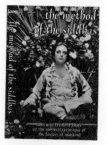

THE METHOD
OF THE SIDDHAS
Talks with Franklin Jones on
the Spiritual Technique
of the Saviors of Mankind
$3.95

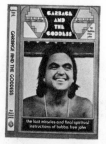

GARBAGE AND
THE GODDESS
The Last Miracles and
Final Spiritual Instructions
of Bubba Free John
$4.95

Order from: The Dawn Horse Communion, Star Route 2, Middletown, Ca. 95461. Include $.35 per book for shipping; Ca. residents add 6% tax.

NO REMEDY: An Introduction to the Life and Practices of the Spiritual Community of Bubba Free John. By Bubba Free John

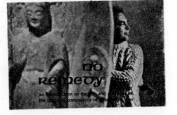

"The primary purpose of this book is to serve as a practical guide for those who have acknowledged Bubba Free John as Guru and joined his community of devotees, The Dawn Horse Communion. It is for those who no longer have any choice but to be undone in God.

"This is not to say that *No Remedy* is useless to the general reader. *On the contrary, anyone genuinely interested in spiritual life cannot help but benefit from this book.* It communicates specific information about the radical sadhana of the Way of Understanding that will certainly illumine (if not undermine) one's knowledge of spiritual practices in general. It is rich with the humor of a path that is free of dilemma and assumed difficulty from beginning to end. And, besides outlining the basic conditions and practices of this sadhana, *No Remedy* presents Bubba Free John's incisive commentary on pertinent topics ranging from homosexuality to dietary fanaticism to the politics of the spiritual community." —from the Preface

$3.50

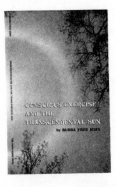

CONSCIOUS EXERCISE AND THE TRANSCENDENTAL SUN. By Bubba Free John

Conscious exercise is not a matter of muscle-building or of motivated purification of the body for "spiritual" ends. As Bubba Free John notes in this detailed, illustrated instructional guide for his Ashram, conscious exercise is a happy and humorous responsibility for those already assuming the Divine as their present condition. It is direct participation in the process of conducting the life-force from and to its Divine Source through simple, balanced movements and natural breathing.

$1.95

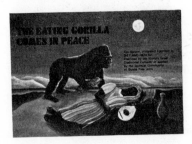

THE EATING GORILLA COMES IN PEACE. By Bubba Free John

This book, which is the basic guide to the lacto-vegetarian diet and the health practices required of all members of The Dawn Horse Communion, undermines all conventional approaches to diet and the search for Truth via "lunch." It discusses the natural and intelligent management of diet and health as a functional condition for sadhana, or right action in relationship with the Guru. When the search for "cure" (or perfect body or perfect health) is obviated, then the body may be purified and brought naturally into functional harmony.

Order from: The Dawn Horse Communion, Star Route 2, Middletown, Ca. 95461. Include $.35 per book for shipping; Ca. residents add 6% tax.

$3.50

THE DAWN HORSE: Critical and challenging forums to promote real understanding of the great traditions of esoteric spirituality. Published bi-monthly by The Dawn Horse Communion as a basic instrument of the Teaching of the Dharma of Understanding, the magazine presents and discusses other teachings and practices in relation to that Dharma as taught by Bubba Free John. Each issue features a theme like "Four Forms of Buddhism," "Healing and Magic," "Esotericism in the Middle Eastern Religions," or "Transpersonal Psychology" —interviews and articles by leading spiritual authorities such as Lama Govinda,

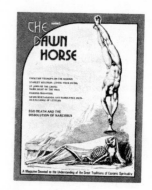

Chogyam Trungpa Rinpoche, and Pir Vilayat Khan—profiles on Ramana Maharshi, Shirdi Sai Baba, Anandamayi Ma, St. Seraphim of Sarov, Hui Neng (the 6th Zen Patriarch), and other Masters—reprints from the best, most provocative traditional and contemporary literature, like the classic *Lankavatara Sutra* and Meher Baba's *Listen, Humanity*. And, the original essays and talks of Bubba Free John. Through provocative, in-depth statements and commentary, *The Dawn Horse* seeks to illumine the real assumptions, processes, and realizations of the esoteric traditions of man.

Subscriptions: $15 for six issues (postpaid); $3 for single copies ($.35 for shipping). Order from: The Dawn Horse Communion, Star Route 2, Middletown, Ca. 95461.

THE GORILLA SERMON: A Record Album of Talks by Bubba Free John on the Radical Nature of Spiritual Life.

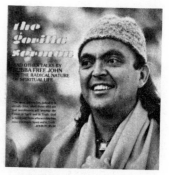

Bubba Free John is a contemporary Man of Understanding, a perfectly awakened being, who speaks and acts from a point of view that is radical, and perhaps disturbing to the conventional mind. *THE GORILLA SERMON* is a two-record collection of excerpts from some of the most powerful talks Bubba has given to his devotees.

"A great teacher with a dynamic ability to awaken in his listeners something of the Divine Reality in which he is grounded, with which he is identified and which in fact he is."

—Israel Regardie

$5.98. Order from: The Dawn Horse Communion, Star Route 2, Middletown, Ca. 95461. Include $.50 per record for shipping. Ca. residents add 6% tax.

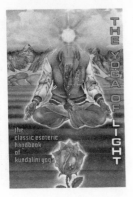

THE YOGA OF LIGHT
The Classic Esoteric
Handbook of Kundalini Yoga
By Hans-Ulrich Reiker

Generally acknowledged as a classic, this ancient text is a primary traditional source on the functional relationship between the intuited Divine Reality and the life-process which is always proceeding directly from it.

"Our endeavor here is not so much to enrich science as a to enrich ourselves, and he who enriches his self, his inner Self, does he not also enrich the science of man?" — Hans-Ulrich Reiker

$3.95

THE SPIRITUAL INSTRUCTIONS OF SAINT SERAPHIM OF SAROV
Edited and with an introduction by Bubba Free John

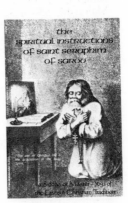

An extraordinary account of the sadhana and realized spirituality of the great 19th century Russian Siddha. An introduction and life by A. F. Dobbie-Bateman is followed by the famous "Conversation" of Seraphim with Nicholas Motovilov. The Holy Spirit or Maha Shakti was powerfully alive in Saint Seraphim, and the text describes direct transmission of his spiritual consciousness and force.

$1.95

THE SONG OF THE SELF SUPREME
(Astavakra Gita)
Translated by Radhakamal Mukerjee

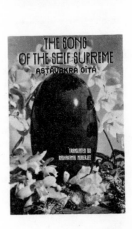

Few ancient treatises show such profound and lively concern with the ultimate reality. It presents Astavakra's teaching, based upon the Upanisadic creed of absolute monism, in the form of a dialogue with Janaka, the seer-king of Videha. This translation brings the true meaning of this illustrious Vedantic text to light for the first time for English readers and establishes it as one of the greatest texts in the history of spiritual literature.

$3.95

Order from: The Dawn Horse Communion, Star Route 2, Middletown, Ca 95461. Include $.35 per book for shipping; Ca. residents add 6% tax.